Native American Herbal Healing Apothecary

Learn How to Use the Herbs and Plants of North America as Medicine

Grow a Healing Herb Garden, Wildcrafting, Foraging, to Heal Any Ailment

By

Brianna Claymore

Publishing House

Cover design

Lisa Cunningham

First Edition

Contents

Special Thanks

I must extend a very special thank you to my dear friend Grace Blackrock. As you'll read, it was her deep knowledge of herbal remedies that first sparked my interest.

I would also like to thank Steve "Little Wolf" Countryman for answering so many endless questions that I had as I was writing this book. Thank you!

Also, I would like to thank you, the reader. Without your support in purchasing this book, I would not be able to sustain my emerging writing career.

Would you do me a huge favor? Would you kindly leave a review where you purchased this book online? I would really appreciate it.

An Interest in Alternatives

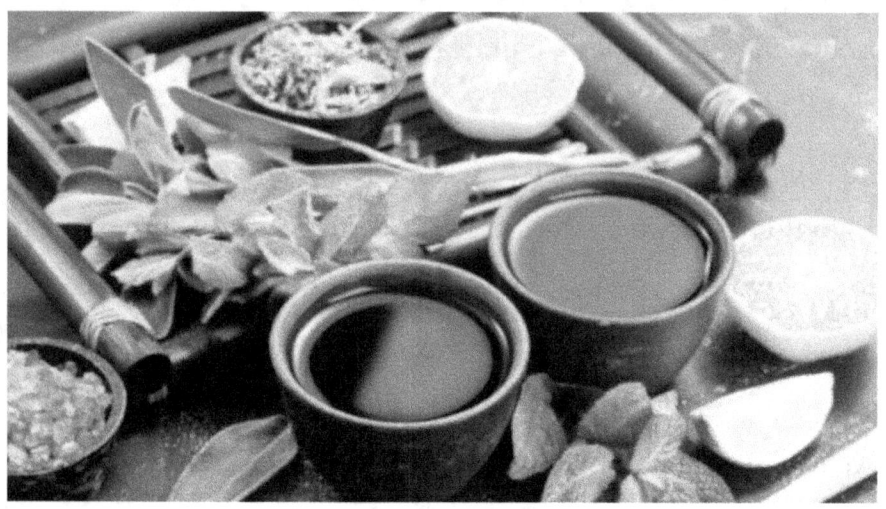

"We have forgotten how to heal ourselves."

Those are the words of my life-long friend, Grace. They resonate with me to this day, even though she has been gone for decades.

I was no more than seven years old when I first met her. My family moved into the house next door to her. I would see her in the back of her house, in a large field, bending over and picking flowers. That's what my child's mind saw. I finally got the courage to speak to her. That was the day Grace changed my life.

She treated me as if I were her own granddaughter. I learned she was Native American. In my young mind, it conjured up all sorts of exotic images. But I had no idea the herbal knowledge she held within her.

I trudged with her throughout the field as she selected certain plants and dug them up or picked off flower petals or leaves. She would tell me how each plant could help heal a part of the body.

Grace loved stinging nettles, she said, because it eased her arthritis. "My grandmother taught me the value of this plant for my joints." Then she said, "My ancestors used this for headaches as well."

As she told me about what I thought were the magical properties of these plants, she would say, "We have forgotten to heal ourselves."

The Cost is Too High

"Modern medicine is great, don't get me wrong," she told me once, as we sat in her house as she prepared a tea from the herbs we just picked. "When necessary, I use it myself. But the price sometimes is too high for me."

When I was younger, I didn't completely understand what she meant by that, but I filed it away because I found all of her words to be wise. I knew one day I would.

As my friendship with Grace matured, I found out she was not only an herbalist, immersed in the traditions of her Native American culture, but she was a nurse. As we walked through the fields one day, she stopped at a specific plant and bent down to pick its leaves. "A patient of mine had an allergic reaction to a medicine today," she said, "but this --" she waved the leaves – "this will do the same thing." She paused a beat. "Without doing harm."

I went home that day and thought about Grace. Up until that moment, I saw her as a Native American who stubbornly clung to her "old ways." When I discovered, however, she was a nurse, an occupation in which she used allopathic medicine, then something clicked in my mind.

The two branches of healing weren't in conflict as I had always thought. They could live together in harmony. I considered our society's dependence on not only prescription medication but over-the-counter drugs as well. The more I thought, the more I knew that herbal healing could help us. After doing some research, I discover that nearly two million people a year have adverse reactions to prescription drugs serious enough to send them to the hospital. That is an astoundingly large number.

Did other people know this? And if they did, why are they so complacent about it? Grace's words again echoed in my head: the price is sometimes too high. This is what she was talking about.

Capturing an Oral Tradition

That was the moment when I realized exactly how the practice of herbalism could help us. Native American herbs – the ones Grace taught me to use and respect --

offer us an alternative. I vowed that others needed to know more about herbalism and its benefits. If through her knowledge, even one person was saved from a severe reaction to a pharmaceutical, it was worth it.

While I always paid attention to Grace when we were on our field trips, I was now seized with a passion and drive to record her herbal knowledge. It's no exaggeration that for nearly a millennial or more, Native Americans have passed down these teachings orally. There was no herbal handbook Grace consulted. It was all in her head.

I felt a sense of urgency to record this, not only so Grace's words would be remembered, and I could learn from her, but so others could also explore the possibility of a gentler, kinder form of healing. I took everything she knew and wrote it down. I visited her daily. We grew closer. With every visit, my passion grew for this more natural form of health.

But my education didn't end with Grace's field lessons and long talks. I've since gathered everything I could learn about Native American herbs and added to her near-encyclopedic knowledge. I've traveled the country and interviewed individuals with Native American heritage who were willing to share their herbal secrets with me. And I tag-teamed that knowledge – which otherwise was in danger of being lost – with what the contemporary researchers discovered about these herbs.

The result? This volume of more than 50 of the most effective herbs from Native American culture and folklore. Within the pages of this book, you'll find these natural remedies categorized by their healing properties. Got a headache? Then look under that heading to find the natural remedies that not only the Native Americans used but are also verified scientifically to help. If you have an arthritis flare-up and don't want to reach for the mega-strength drug, look it up here to find a safer way to extinguish the pain.

You'll not only discover which herbs are the most effective for your health condition, but which is the best way to use them as well as for instructions. You'll learn the difference between an infusion and a paste and be able to create them for you and your family.

How to Use this Book

But this book is more – much more – than just a guide to herbal usage. You'll also get a snapshot of Native American culture. Did you know that they had rituals and ceremonies that accompanied their healing practices, which reflected their holistic beliefs? In the first few chapters of this guidebook, you'll learn about them as well as their holistic approach to life.

How did they choose the proper herbs and ensure they didn't deplete their supply? They used a method that today we call wildcrafting. You'll learn the method and even get instructions on how to do it responsibly.

I also provide you with a short, comprehensive review of the history of herbalism. We'll talk about the growing profession of herbalists and what that entails in today's increasingly technological age. I've also included thorough instructions for making your own tinctures, pastes, and other applications of these seemingly miraculous plants.

Hopefully, this book will ignite your own passion for herbal healing. If that's the case, then you'll be pleased to learn that Part Three describes how you can be your own herbalist. From wildcrafting – the responsible approach to herbal gathering – to the drying of the plants and their proper storage, it's an inclusive beginner's guide to home herbal healing.

Don't worry if you're not familiar with some of the terms used in this book. I explain them all when I introduce them, but I also included an easy-to-use glossary for your reference. Whether you're new to the herbalist tradition and especially that of the Native Americans or if you're a veteran herbalist, you'll find something new about herbs and herbal healing here.

This book represents only a part of my life-long learning about herbal healing. I'm still on my journey that began when Grace shared her Native American knowledge with me. I like to believe Grace would be proud of this book.

Chapter 1: Why Herbal Medicine

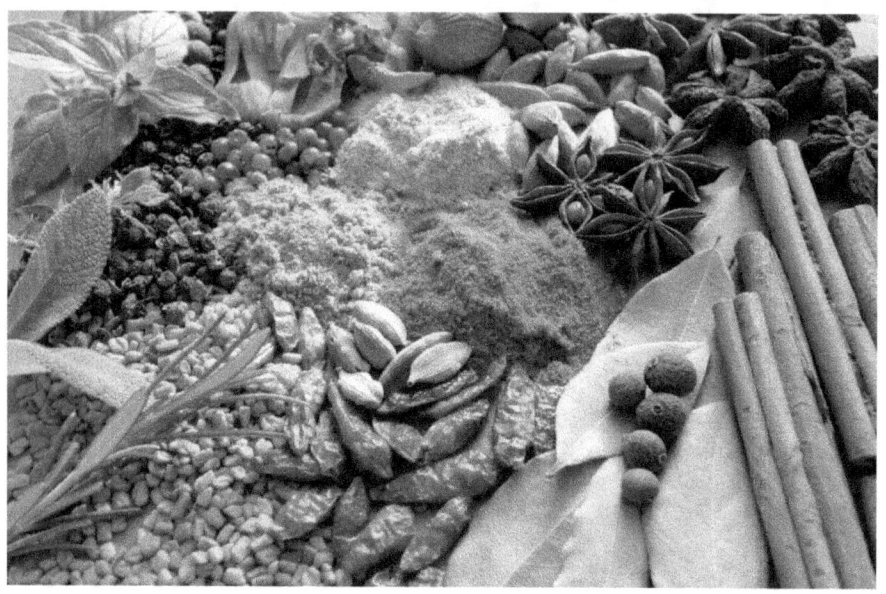

In an age when we can cure or at least alleviate nearly every ailment under the sun with a quick trip to the drug store or a rapid prescription process, why bother with herbal healing?

Thanks to the miraculous advances of allopathic medicine in the twentieth century and beyond, we take for granted that we have more ways to alleviate even our most stubborn pain and ease, if not cure, the symptoms of diseases that killed our grandparents and even our parents.

Why not take advantage of the miraculous new pharmaceuticals available to us?

Those are questions I get asked frequently. Surprisingly, my answer is: of course, you should. We would be silly not to use them when appropriate. But, as my friend, Grace, constantly reminded me, there is a price that comes with the march of progress.

Every person who uses herbal healing has their own reasons for doing so. But underlying these personal preferences are some excellent arguments.

The Botanical Origin of Medications

It surprises many individuals to learn that nearly half of today's pharmaceuticals exist due to the healing ability of an herb. Whether it was an observant Alexander Fleming who noticed the antibiotic properties of mold or the Jesuits who witnessed the power of the Cinchona calisaya tree in treating malaria, observations like this ignited the creation of the pharmaceutical.

Armed with that knowledge, scientists then extracted the active ingredient from the plant and used it as the basis of prescription medication. If we can get all the benefits of these herbs with a simple pill or injection, why go through all the trouble of cultivating, harvesting herbs?

But are we really getting the full potency of the herb? The pharmaceutical industry wants us to believe we are all packaged conveniently in a capsule or pill. Or in isolating what we know is the active ingredient, are we missing out on a fuller, more robust healing? Herbalists believe we are. And so does Dr. Andrew Weil.

This isolation of the active chemical works in theory and produces potent and successful medications. But as Weil and herbalists point out, plants possess a large variety of chemical compounds. These compounds work together to create a synergistic effect that may often be more potent than a pill, which contains a single compound of the plant.

Weil believes in the synergy of the full herb. Every time

researchers pluck an active ingredient from the plant and isolate it for a drug, Dr. Weil believes the ingredient becomes less effective. The synergy is lost.

The extraction procedure, while beneficial, bypasses a large portion of the true healing power of the plant, he says. He believes that a large part of extracting active chemicals singly has more to do with expediency and profit than treating diseases.

Weil's theory is that pharmaceutical companies are not necessarily run for the greater good. Instead, he thinks this process, however helpful it is to our health, is done for corporate expediency and profits.

The big drug companies carry this strategy out in two ways, the medical doctor and alternative healer says. The first is the simplification of the research process. Isolating what appears to be the active ingredient and discarding the rest of the plant makes for quick development.

And this brings us to the second way. The faster pharmaceutical companies can develop effective medications, the more profits they can generate.

Selling Drugs in America

It's true that pharmaceutical companies need to make money, and we, as consumers, need their products at times. But consider this: the American public spent $369.7 billion on prescription medications in 2019, an increase of 5.7% from the previous year.

That didn't happen by chance. The drug companies spend big bucks to make sure not only your doctor is aware of all the latest and (supposedly) greatest medications to treat every condition, but you're aware of them as well.

In fact, the pharmaceuticals collectively spend $3 billion yearly promoting their wares to you and me. They also spend another $24 billion in marketing to health care professionals.

The most alarming part of this information shouldn't be the amount of money spent on advertising, but the fact drug companies can advertise at all. In every other country except New Zealand, there are no direct-to-consumer advertising of prescription drugs. It's illegal in every other country on the planet.

You should ask yourself: How many patients – or as the drug companies think of us, consumers – are swayed by the commercials? How many people head straight to their doctors to ask for the latest and greatest drug? That's exactly what the pharmaceutical industry wants you to do.

There's still another, perhaps even more important, question you need to ask: Is my health care provider swayed by the promotions and giveaways of the drug salesmen? Is he prescribing my family drugs we don't really need?

Years ago, I took my then six-year-old daughter to the doctor for mild illness. Her doctor told me he would write a prescription if I insisted, but he was sure the problem would go away on its own. I declined the drug. But it aroused my curiosity. Would all doctors give the patient a choice like that? And perhaps even more concerning: How many patients feel if they don't walk out of their doctor's office with a prescription in hand, then their doctor didn't do their job?

Herbal Healing Advantages

As the general public embraced the advancement of the allopathic method and especially of the breakthrough drug treatments, herbal healing took a back seat. Not only was it shunned by many, but its efficacy was also questioned.

But that's all changing. It's difficult to find statistics on herbal use alone, but a recent government study indicated up to one-third of the population use some form of alternative therapies.

There are many reasons for their popularity. Herbal remedies are far more affordable than conventional medicine and more accessible. But perhaps its greatest strength is that it balances your system. The phytonutrients contribute to the stabilization of your hormones and your metabolism. And unlike conventional drugs, which may drain your immune system, many herbs actually boost your immunity.

Instead of passively accepting prescription after prescription, the larger question we all should answer for our own health and wellbeing is how many prescriptions are too many? Is every prescription you're taking necessary? Are there alternatives to those over-the-counter medications you take?

The Native American approach to illness is holistic. If you have a cough or a cold, the herbal remedy doesn't treat only the symptom; it treats you as a person. The herb rebalances your mind, body, and spirit. That according to their philosophy, this is true healing.

Native Americans were successful herbal healers for centuries. And today, their remedies remain just as effective. That's the ultimate reason Native American herbal healing is growing in popularity. There are statistics to prove this.

Of the ten herbs used most in the United States, seven of them come from Native Americans. That speaks volumes on the efficacy of the Native American's ability to heal with herbs.

The Importance of Phytonutrients

For those of you still debating the efficacy of herbs, let's look at these plants a bit deeper. They all have one thing in common that enables them to work their seemingly miraculous healings. They all contain phytonutrients.

Phytonutrients, or phytochemicals, are natural compounds found in all plants. The name is derived from the Greek word for plant, *phyto*. Their first task is to protect the plant from insects, fungi, germs, and other adversaries. Not only that but plant all plant-based food also contains these crucial substances, including whole grains, nuts, beans, and tea.

Scientists have been able to identify more than 25,000 of these chemicals. Modern medicine has also discovered that phytonutrients contain healing properties. They have antimicrobial, antibacterial, and anticancer agents. They contain chemicals that help to alleviate inflammation.

Take, for example, garlic. Its main active ingredient is allicin, the chemical that gives it that characteristic strong odor. But this same chemical also makes this herb a powerful tool in fighting bacteria and viruses.

That's not the only active healing substance in this plant. It has nearly 30 other active substances. The beneficial effects of allicin only last a mere three hours, but as a consequence of that chemical's breakdown, more healing chemicals are produced.

The healing properties of herbs are an intricate balance of all of their phytonutrients. This brings us full circle to Dr. Weil's idea that by isolating the active ingredient, we lose something of its full medicinal effects. But then, the Native Americans knew that all along.

Properly practiced herbal medicine can offer you a natural, safer, and holistic avenue on your path to a healthier, happier life.

Chapter 2: What is Herbalism?

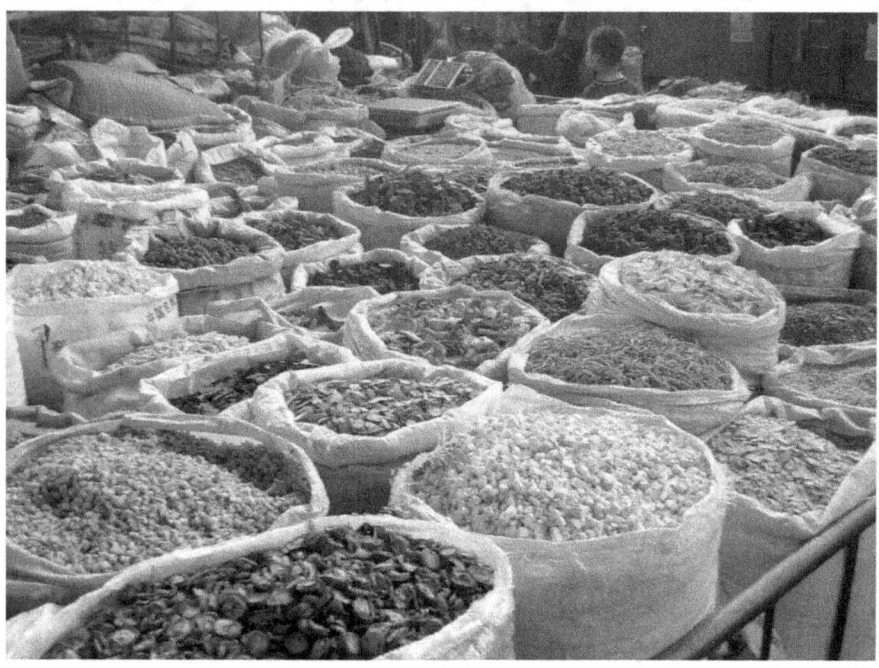

Herbalism, which many call phytotherapy, is the use of plants for healing as well as for the maintenance of good health. It is the oldest known medical practice. Before doctors were able to employ synthetic prescription drugs, they used what they had at hand: plants. It is, in fact, the most widely used form of medicine on the planet. More than 80 percent of the world's population employ it even today.

Perhaps the major tenet of herbalism that separates it from conventional Western medicine is its holistic nature. Unlike pharmaceuticals, which use isolated compounds from the plants, herbalism employs the entire plant. This is vital since herbalists believe that the substances of the herb are naturally balanced. Using them in that state only encourages healing of the body, mind, and spirit.

The herbalist or herbal therapist, as those who practice this tradition, are called, focus on individual therapy. When recommending herbs and treatments, the goal is to incorporate all aspects of the person's life, including mental, emotional, spiritual realms, as well as the social and environmental areas.

Good health, according to the herbal tradition, is more than merely the absence of disease. It is the existence of a positive state of wellbeing. Herbalism advocates and strives for the promotion of health, certainly. But in contrast to conventional medicine, its goal is to prevent the disease in the first place.

To this end, the herbal healer and the person seeking healing are active partners in the endeavor. The herbalist provides his "patient" with the tools that will spark his body's innate ability to heal itself. Unlike that of conventional medicine, where a patient waits to be treated and cured by the physician, herbalism places the role of healing directly in the individual's hands.

Herbal medicine is misunderstood by many because it blurs the line between foods and medicines, according to Dr. Andrew Weil. Of course, this is why so many of us are interested in it. And this is why the modern medical community – especially the FDA – doesn't quite know what to do with it.

The FDA – the Food and Drug Administration – is tasked with ensuring all medicines meet stringent safety requirements. Part of that process is the reviewing of massive amounts of research as well as reviews of human trials of the drug or vaccine.

Herbs escape this intense scrutiny. And so, the FDA has no record of clinical research on them, no human scientific trials, and no way to issue an edict on them. Unlike what some in the medical community may tell you, that doesn't mean the use of herbs is unsafe. There may not but clinical evidence of it its effectiveness, but there is abundant anecdotal evidence.

And here's a quirk in the system. If tests were done on a certain herb, and the FDA would sanction its use, the herb would immediately be classified as a drug. When someone warns you about herbal use due to no FDA sanction, remember this.

Herbal healing predates the FDA and modern medicine by literal eons. It is, without a doubt, the oldest healing practice on the planet; its use dating back to thousands of years. The use of plants for medicinal purposes is far older than recorded history. Archeologists have discovered the use of plants for this purpose as far back as the Paleolithic age, about 60,000 years ago. (Curiously, humans weren't the first to discover this practice. It seems that other primates also used herbs to treat their illnesses.)

Every culture has its own system of herbal medicine based on its own cultural mores and the plants available in the region.

Ayurvedic Medicine

One of the most well-known herbal systems – and one of the oldest -- is that of India, called Ayurveda. Some believe the use of this particular system of healing began as early as 4,000 BC. The basis of this knowledge is in no small part based on the earliest Sanskrit texts, including the Rig Veda and the Atharva Veda.

Nearly 20 percent of the population of the Indian subcontinent uses some form of this system of medicine that emphasizes the personalization of treatment. Deepak Chopra is its most recognized proponent. A trained medical doctor, he also advocates for the natural, holistic healing of Ayurveda.

Chinese Herbalism

China's traditional system of medicine is also familiar to many and used far outside the boundaries of that country. It has given westerners acupuncture and acupressure. In addition, though, the Chinese have developed a sophisticated system of herbs. The herbs are but a part of what is called Traditional Chinese Medicine. The Chinese, just like the Native Americans, believe that healing an illness is a holistic endeavor. Ailments are a sign your body is out of balance. Traditional Chinese Medicine views the balance of life as two opposing energy forces, the yin, and the yang.

In addition, they believe that the entire world – the universe, in fact – is made of five elements: fire, earth, metal, and wood. The herbs used for healing are not surprisingly categorized into five tastes: sweet, salty, bitter, pungent, and sour, which correspond to the elements.

Western Herbalism

There is an herbal healing tradition in the Western Hemisphere as well, even though allopathic medicine has tried to reduce it to second class status and seems at times to try to discredit. It. The ancient Greeks and Romans relied on herbs.

The schism in western medicine of modern medicine and herbal healing may have first begun with Hippocrates. You no doubt have heard of the Hippocratic oath doctors take, but his influence goes beyond that.

He is credited with the authorship of a text called Hippocratic Corpus, which includes herbal recipes and remedies. Inside the pages of this text, there are countless herbs not only native to Greece but also from other geographical areas. It is a very complete compendium.

While the information is nearly identical to what religious healers were using at the time, there is one big difference. Hippocrates didn't include the ceremonies and rituals that accompanied those remedies. This omission reveals the logic and the reason with which he approached his vocation.

Herbalism of the Middle Ages

The primary source of all medical knowledge in Europe during the middle ages resided within the Benedictine monasteries. It's been noted that most of the herbal knowledge they possessed was passed down to them from the Greeks and Romans. In turn, the monks laboriously copied these herbs and their uses so as not to lose them. The abbeys naturally became the repositories of medical knowledge. Their gardens, in addition, grew the plants used in the remedies.

But that doesn't mean that herbal healing wasn't practiced by the common man. Folk medicine, as we have come to call it, continued unabated both in the home and also in the villages. Because of this, you could find either local or itinerant herbalists. The term used to describe these individuals was wise man or woman. They prescribed the remedies, which at times included spells, advice, and what was thought to be divine insight.

One of the most famous wise women was Hildegard of Bingen. A 12th-century Benedictine nun, she composed the legendary medical text Causae et Curae. Hildegard was a remarkable woman whose faith in natural healing came arose from her faith in the Scripture. In this, her beliefs are similar to that of the Native Americans. Her practice was a natural product in the knowledge that mankind as a spiritual creation is not solely bound by natural laws but also a high spiritual law as well. Today, you can find modern European herbalists who still use many of her remedies.

In a very real sense, all the other medical practices that have followed owe a debt of gratitude to the study and use of herbs.

The term herbalism encompasses more than just the use of plants for healing. Many contemporary herbalists practice other approaches to holistic healing, not unlike the Native Americans. Some of their techniques include detoxification, hydrating the body, as well as exercise, and getting outdoors frequently.

The core concept the drives all herbal practice is not only the belief in the healing power of plants but the corollary love of nature and a respect for the environment.

Chapter 3: What Does an Herbalist Do?

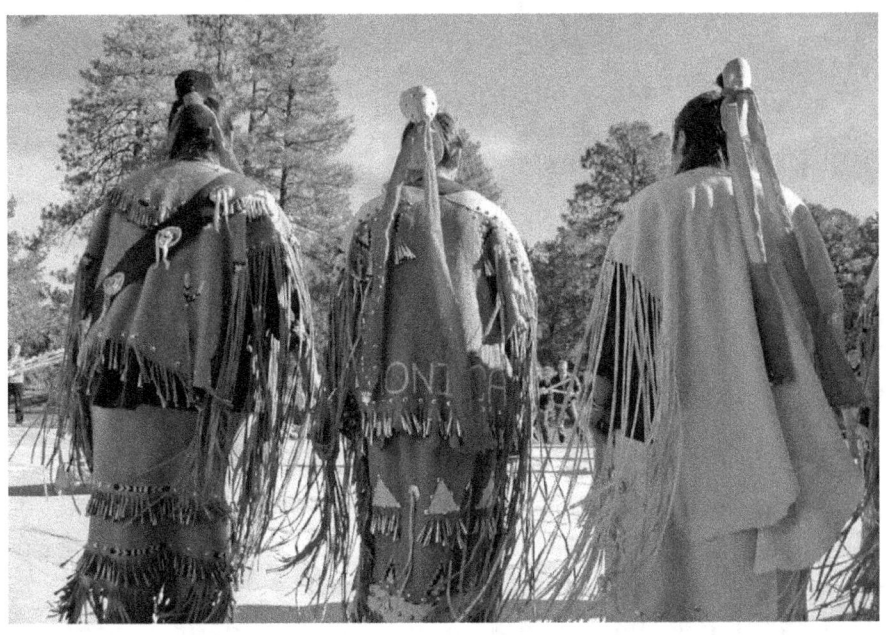

The definition of an herbalist is relatively straightforward. It's a professional trained in the use of herbs and related naturally occurring, plant-derived substances for medicinal purposes. But the duties of a professional herbalist are far more intricate and encompassing.

To start with, an herbalist may specialize in one aspect of

the craft. It may be in the cultivation of the herbs or the harvesting and collecting of plants in the wild. Some herbalists strictly provide appropriate herbal prescriptions and knowledgeable advice. And, of course, many professionals perform all these duties.

The United States has no federal licensing organization for herbalists similar to the American Medical Association for doctors. These professionals are, however, guided and supported by the American Herbalist Guild, which offers a clear outline for its profession. Founded in 1989, the AHG is an educational organization, which promotes education and professionalism in its ranks.

Many colleges that specialize in holistic and alternative medicine offer courses that lead to a certificate or diploma in herbalism, after which you become a master herbalist. As you may guess, these courses include classes in botany and plant science as well as evidence-based botanical research. But they also include courses in anatomy, biochemistry, and physiology, as well as nutrition. In addition, students take coursework in the field of pharmacy and dispensing.

In addition to the variety of course work, any person undergoing a serious degree in herbalism also engages in real-life experiences and clinical memberships. Above and beyond that, there are activities that extend beyond the academic and span their lifetime, some of which are continuing workshops, webinars, and conferences.

If you've never seen an herbalist before, be prepared for it to be different than a visit with your physician or other health care providers. For the most part, if you're like many of us, you see your medical doctor for one reason: your physical health. Seldom do we seek his advice on mental or emotional issues. And when we do, it's usually because those areas affect our physical health.

You can expect your herbalist to initially conduct a clinical exam. They will look at the areas of the body that you're concerned about. If you have a bruise or burn, they'll inspect that, of course.

While your physical health may be the primary reason for plant-based healing, don't expect it to be the only topic your herbalist touches on. In fact, they will touch on three overarching areas, including your physical and emotional wellbeing and your metaphysical environment.

Your herbalist will ask you about the amount of sleep you average, your relationships with your family, your community, and your job. During this time, you may even talk about your spiritual beliefs if you have any.

You're probably already got the idea that an appointment with a professionally trained herbalist isn't going to be a five-minute visit where you tell him what hurts, and he whips out an herb.

The underlying fundamental tenet of herbalism is holism. A professional herbalist will spend time learning about you so they can treat you as a person, not merely treat your symptom. Your relationship with your personal herbalist will not only be beneficial to your physical health, but it will also be good for you mentally and spiritually.

Chapter 4: Native Americans and Herbalism

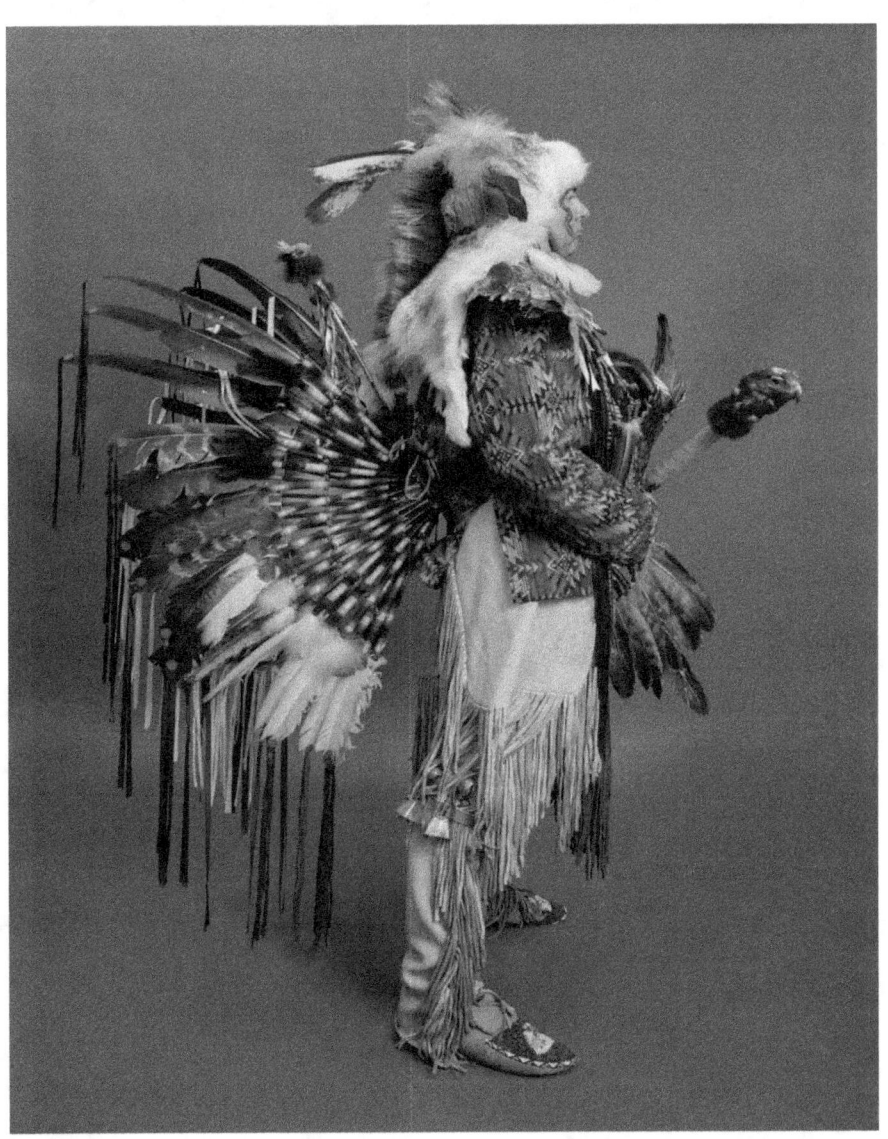

To our western eyes, the Native American legacy may seem like a paradox. Clearly, what we call Native American is a convenient umbrella term that identifies the countless nations and tribes of the indigenous people of North America. Today, the U.S. government recognizes more than 500 of these tribes. Despite the immense diversity in these groups, though, they all honor a common attitude toward not only herbalism but deep, reverential regard for life and all living things.

To more clearly understand their culture, it helps to learn about the areas they inhabited and how they lived. It's impossible in this volume to mention them all, but several of these nations and tribes are well known, and it's from these we have received the wealth of herbal remedies handed down orally from generation to generation. They are identified by the geographical areas they lived. This chapter is a short primer of the tribes organized by their geographical regions.

The Northeast

The Native Americans who inhabited the northeast were the first to meet the European settlers. This geographical region includes the eastern seaboard from Canada to North Carolina and extends inland to the Mississippi Valley.

Two main groups lived here. The first was a group called the Iroquoian speakers and included Cayuga, Erie, Oneida, Onondaga, Seneca, and Tuscarora tribes. The majority of these peoples lived along rivers inland in small villages.

The second group spoke Algonquian. These tribes included Delaware, Fox, Menominee, Pequot, and Shawnee. They were located along the ocean in farming and fishing villages and grew crops.

The Southeast

This area is described by historians as that area north of the Gulf of Mexico and south of the northeast region of North America. The tribes that made this area home were tribes sometimes referred to as the Five Civilized Tribes and included the Cherokee, Chickasaw, Choctaw, Creek, and Seminole. The majority of these individuals spoke a dialect of the Muskogean language.

These people were skilled farmers with a long list of staple crops: beans, maize, squash, sunflower, and tobacco. They organized their society around small ceremonial and market villages called hamlets.

The Plains

The culture which today we call the plains is the vast prairie region west of the Mississippi River to the Rocky Mountains. It's a sprawling area that extends as far north as Canada and as far south as the Gulf of Mexico.

These peoples lived as hunters and farmers. They were also a mixed group of tribes that spoke various languages, including Algonquian, Caddoan, Uto-Aztecan, Athabaskan, and Siouan.

After the Spanish colonists introduced these peoples to the horse, however, they adopted a nomadic life. The tribes that lived in this area, including the Blackfeet Arapaho, Cheyenne, Crow, and Comanche, rode horses and followed the migration of the buffalo across the prairie.

Their home was a teepee, the cone-shaped structure many of us think of as being uniquely Native American. Covered with buffalo skin, this portable structure could be folded and taken with them. This is also the culture that is well known for its feathered headdresses.

The Southwest

The Southwest consisted of the large desert region they called home, including not only what is today Arizona and New Mexico, but portions of Colorado, Utah, and Texas. The area is indeed large and produced two separate cultures.

One culture practiced farming. Tribes like the Hopi, Zuni, Yaqui, and the Yuma grew staple crops, including corn, beans, and squash. They had permanent dwellings, even what could be called apartment complexes. The homes were built out of stone and adobe and had several stories to them. In the center of many of the villages were large ceremonial pit houses called kivas.

The second culture, of which the most well-known are the Navajo and Apache, were nomadic. They hunted and gathered. They also plundered their neighbors, the adobe dwelling tribes, for their crops. These groups are known for their houses, called hogans, which always faced east. These people believed the hogan was gifted to them by the gods and faced it so the family could see the sun as soon as they rose. They were made of mud and bark and less permanent than their neighbors.

The Great Basin

This bowl-like region is bounded by the Rocky Mountains to the east, the Sierra Nevada Mountains to the west, the Columbia Plateau on the north, and on the south by the Colorado Plateau. It's mainly a land of deserts, salt flats, and brackish lakes. Shoshonean and Uto-Aztecan were spoken here by such tribes as the Bannock, Ute, Paiute. They sustained themselves by foraging for roots, seeds, and nuts. They hunted snakes, lizards, and small mammals.

These nomadic people lived in a dwelling called a wikiup, which was made of willow poles or saplings as well as leaves and brush.

California

Even in the sixteenth century, California was a near paradise. With its temperate climate, California boasted a population of 300,000, by far the largest populace on the North American continent.

But this geographical area is also noteworthy for another reason: its diversity. Approximately 100 different tribes and people called it home, with more than 200 dialects spoken.

The languages were derived from various tongues, including the Penutian, the Uto-Aztecan, and Athapaskan. Some of the inhabitants of this area had been driven out of their native homes by the Spaniards who colonized the area east.

Even though they spoke different languages, those who lived in California shared similar lifestyles. They were hunter-gatherers who formed small groups based on family. These became known as tribelets. Relationships among these groups, for the most part, were peaceful.

The Northwest Coast

This region, from British Columbia south to northern California, provided Native Americans with not only a mild climate but with an abundance of natural resources. The obvious advantage was the Pacific Ocean, along with the many rivers in that area. This gave these Native Americans nearly everything they needed. They ate salmon, of course, but they were other fish and shellfish. They even made use of the ocean's sea otters, seals, and whales.

This wealth in raw materials afforded the groups who lived here the luxury of creating permanent villages that boasted populations in the hundreds. Groups that called the Northwest Coast home included many who you may not have heard of. They included the Athapaskan Haida, Tlingit, The Penutian Chinook, Tsimshian, and Coos, as well as the Wakashan and Kwakiutl.

The Plateau

This geographical region is composed of what is today Idaho and Montana as well as eastern Oregon and

Washington. You could find small villages here along the streams and riverbanks where they fished. These indigenous groups also were also hunter-gatherers.

To the south, the people spoke languages that were Penutian in origin. These included the Modoc, Nez Perce, Walla Walla, and Yakima tribes. Their southern counterparts spoke mainly forms of Salishan dialects. These groups included the Skitswish, also known as Coeur d'Alene, and the Salish.

These people were introduced to the horse, but it was through other Native Americans, not European settlers. Using this animal helped them to achieve a greater hunting area as well as enabling them to become traders and messengers between the Northwest and the Plains peoples.

Native Americans Healing Beliefs

Herbalism, as practiced by the Native Americans, is far more than just the dispensation of herbs for isolated symptoms. We've briefly mentioned the culture's belief in healing all areas of the individual: the body, mind, and spirit. But their holistic approach doesn't end with the person's health. Their concept of holism extends to every area of their lives.

I've used the term healing herbs in this volume and referred to the plants and trees that way throughout this book. Native Americans would argue with my term, for they believe that healing isn't the goal at all. The goal is the achievement of a general state of complete wellness. It encompasses more than mere symptoms and physical issues. Wellness is a much broader and more robust condition than mere healing.

The Native American concept of wellness extends to their communities.

Knowing this fundamental concept may help you better understand that the indigenous peoples of North America – for all their differences – took a holistic approach to health that included areas we might not consider related to our wellbeing. They knew the vital importance of their core beliefs, their spirituality, the norms of their communities, and their values. It's the one overarching concept which binds all tribes and nations together.

It's not difficult to see, then, how indigenous cultures embrace nature and honor its rules, and care for the environment. This view is literally limitless, as the Native Americans see the universe as a living entity with creation as a living process. With that mindset, they easily feel a close relationship to all things.

It's vital, then, that they live within nature, not trying to conquer it but to co-exist harmoniously with it. This way of life is seen in their tradition. Rooted in time and in seasons, these practices provide a mindful approach to moving through the year and promote wholeness.

The Native Americans' great sense of gratitude to Mother Nature can be seen in all of their traditions, of which herbalism is merely one. Traditions such as prayerful ceremonies focus on the community's mind, body, and spirit.

Healing Ceremonies

Every Native American tribe conducted healing ceremonies. While the exact activities during these may differ, they all had a common mission: to create balance and harmony in a person's life. These sacred actions sought to help the person acquire a healthier view of their life. The specific type of ceremony depended on the individual and their unique needs. The tools with which they may treat the person with herbs, prayers, or encouraging changes in the way they live.

But it may also mean the performing of a sweat lodge ceremony. The individual would go into a hut filled with steam from the pouring of hot water onto rocks. The goal was to sweat out toxins, and negative energy that they believed were responsible for the imbalance in his life.

Sometimes the best therapy was a vision quest, in which the individual sought to meet with a guardian spirit or an animal spirit for advice and protection.

Another ceremony is the burning of herbs, so they waft throughout the area. Even today, many of us burn sage to protect our homes and clear negativity.

Implementing these various therapies involved a variety of tools, not the least of which was music and sacred chanting. The elder or medicine man of the tribe would chant. Others would beat a steady rhythm on drums and medicine rattles. These two instruments were of vital importance to the healing process. The sounds and rhythm of these are considered to be Mother Earth's heartbeat. Participants in the ceremony would dance in rhythm to the drumbeat, tapping their feet on the ground to every beat of the Earth's heart. It was more than calming and relaxing; it connected them with the Earth.

Other Tools

There were several other healing instruments the Native Americans employed. These tools were used not only during public gatherings but at home in private ceremonies as well.

They regularly consulted animal totems during their sacred ceremonies to learn the wishes of the animal spirits and seek guidance from them. If you've ever used a dream catcher, then you know its purpose. It's used to catch our nightmares through the restoration of the balance of our body, mind, and spirit.

Another vital ceremonial tool is a smudge stick. This is a

small stick or ribbon bound with herbs that are easily carried. The bundle is opened during a ceremony where the necessary amount of the herbs is administered then reclosed. While the herbs vary depending on the region of the Native American groups, most commonly, they're made of some combination of milkweed, echinacea, and wild ginger, elder, sage, and wheatgrass.

Chapter 5: Encyclopedia of Native American Herbal Healing by Condition

"Everything on the Earth has a purpose, every disease an herb to cure it and every person a mission. This is the Indian theory of existence." - Cristal Quintasket

You've decided to make a change in your life and explore new natural methods of healing your body – and even mind and spirit. This section of the book is your partner in your improving your health, boosting your vitality, and adopting a new, more positive look on life.

You don't necessarily need to adopt the entire Native American lifestyle to benefit from herbal healing. One step in the right direction will make a vast difference in your life. To that end, this Native American herbal guide will be an essential tool.

You'll find herbal remedies used by Native Americans listed by the ailment. After a brief discussion of the problem, you'll go on to read the several plants that provide relief and the area of the continent it grows naturally in case you decide to forage herbs yourself. And, of course, the method of preparation is also included.

You'll discover not only that an ailment may be healed with various herbs, but you'll also learn that a single herb can be a remedy for a variety of ailments. Some of these remedies come with warnings. Women who are breastfeeding or pregnant should not use some of them, and several herbs should not be used with certain medications. If you have known allergies to any of these plants, then you shouldn't use them.

I strongly urge you to visit your personal health care provider before you use any of the herbs. This is especially true if you're on any medications treating the disease or ailment for which the herb remedies.

Are you ready to take your first step to robust health, greater vitality, and a renewed love of life?

Acne

Aloe Vera

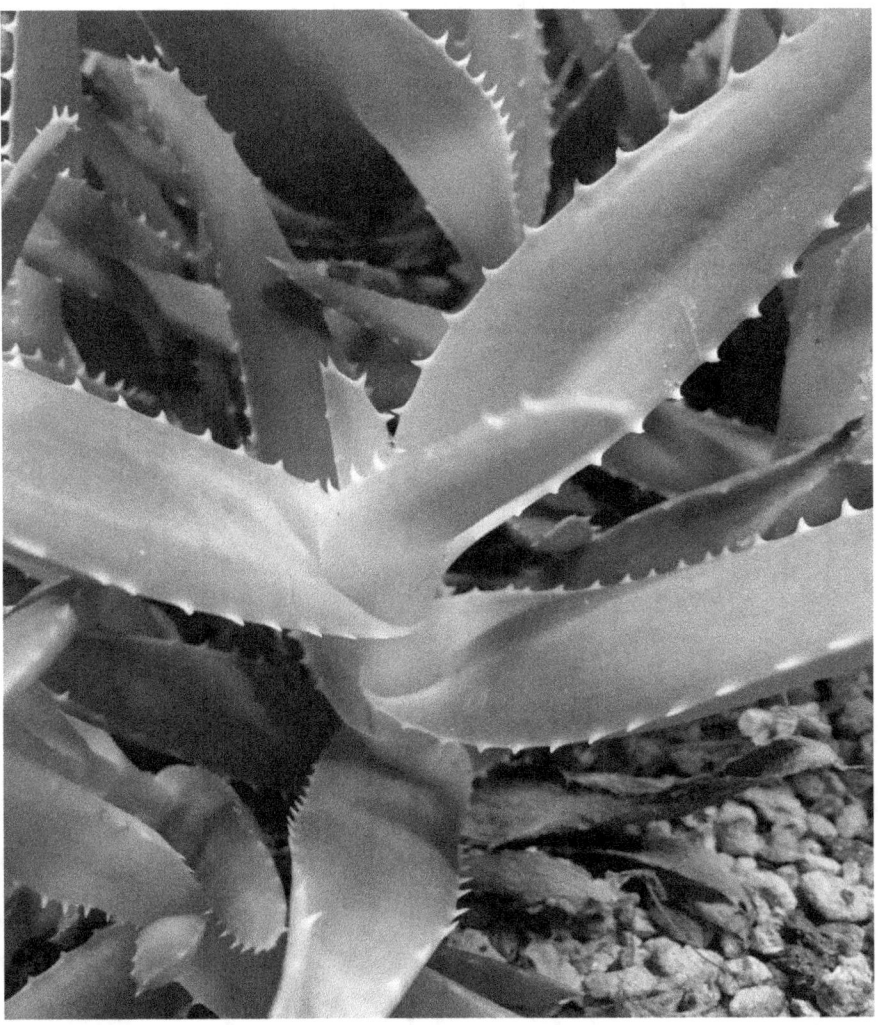

This plant is a remarkable remedy for nearly any skin

problem you may have. It comes as no surprise that it's also an excellent remedy for acne as well.

It has anti-inflammatory and antibacterial properties. Using Aloe Vera is nearly a guarantee that the acne will be less noticeable and your outbreaks fewer.

How to Use: Use the aloe vera gel – straight from the plant if you can – and apply it to the acne. Rinse the area first with warm water. If the fresh herb is unavailable, then you can use a commercial rinse. Just ensure that it contains a minimum of ten percent natural gel.

Basil

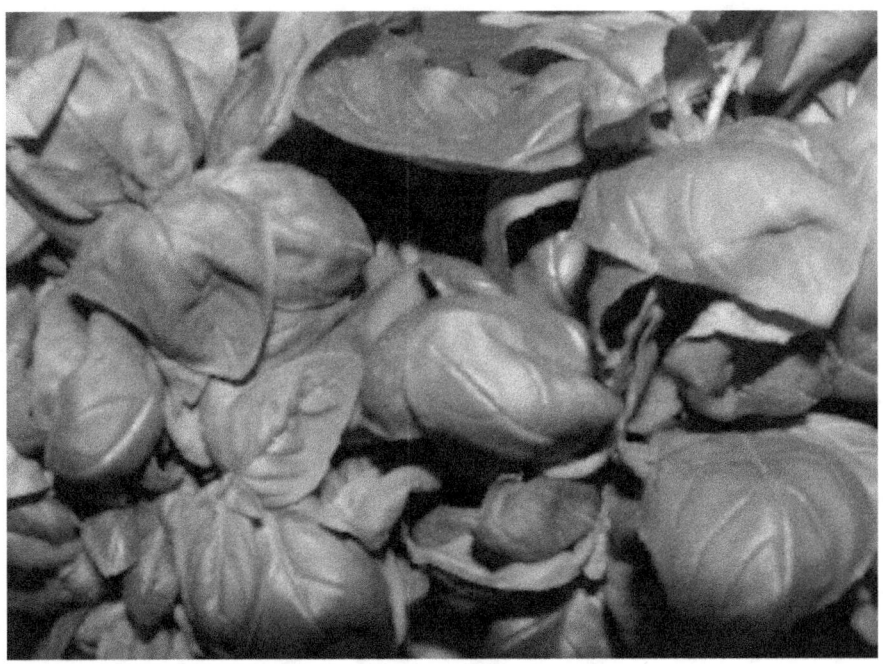

That herb that may either be in your garden or in your windowsill herb box may become the best weapon in your fight against the stubbornness of acne. Why? Because science has determined that basil is an even better astringent than alcohol.

That makes it an excellent asset for managing oil production.

How to Use: Take some stems – you could crush them if you like – and spread them on the area. You can also make a poultice or a salve.

Echinacea

Best known for its ability to boost the immune system, Echinacea also contains anti-inflammatory properties perfect for lessening the swelling around the pimples. Echinacea sounds exotic, but it's nothing more than the coneflower.

This coarse, rough-hairy plant can be found in the prairies, meadows, and woods from the central to the southeastern US.

How to Use: Make a poultice or a salve out of any portion of the plant. Many herbalists, though, believe its root is the most potent.

Garlic

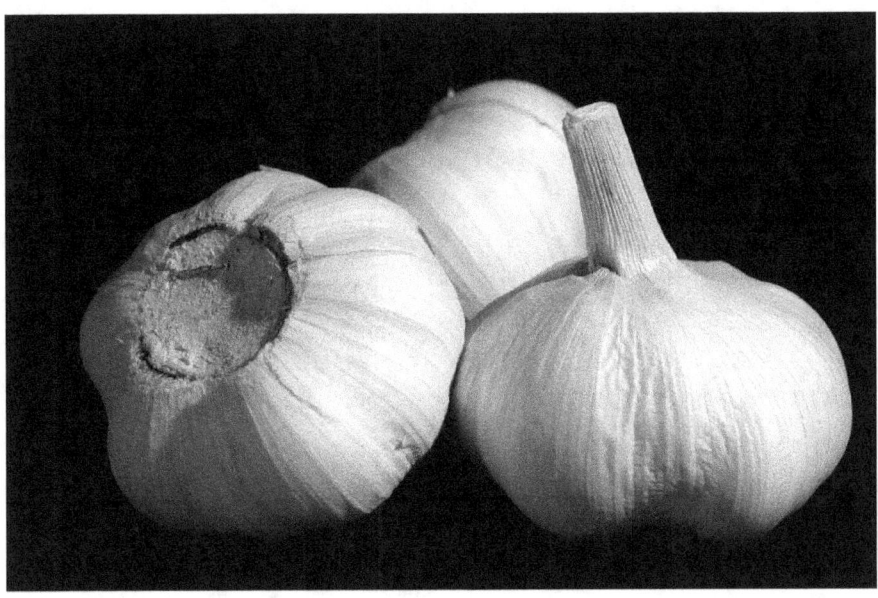

This humble herb, which adds interest to just about every meal, is also very good at healing acne. Its natural anti-inflammatory and antibacterial properties are integral to its powers.

How to Use: Either a poultice or salve or simply add more to your diet.

Honey

As crazy and sticky as this may sound, honey is one of

those wonder ingredients. Not exactly an herb, to be sure, but it was used extensively by the Native Americans as a natural remedy.

Honey is packed with plenty of nutrients and is especially helpful in alleviating acne due to its antioxidants. These are said to help cleanse the pores of waste and debris.

How to Use: Take some honey – local honey, if possible – and dab some on a cotton ball, then gently rub it onto the pimples. You can also make a face mask of the substance.

Jojoba

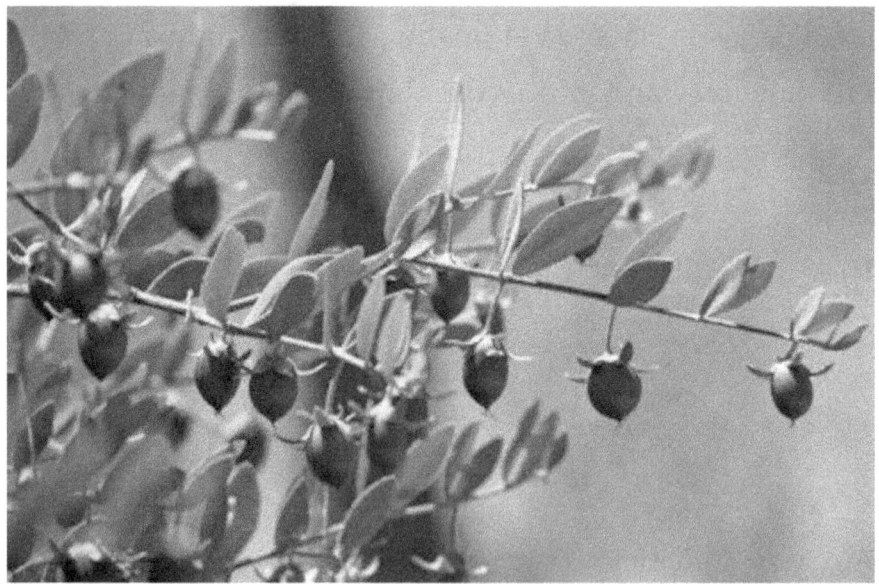

The oil of this plant, found in the arid regions of the southwest of America, has been used for centuries by Native Americas for all types of skin issues, even acne. The reason it works is that the plant's oil contains compounds that aid in lessening skin inflammation, especially those around pimples and whiteheads.

The chances are good that if you don't live near a desert, it'll be difficult to get fresh jojoba oil. But don't worry, because the essential oil of this plant works just as well.

How to Use: Simply blend the oil with a clay face mask cream or gel. Place it on the affected area. An easier and just as effective method of using this remedy is by dabbing a few drops of the oil on a cotton ball and massage the acned area.

Allergies

Garlic

Surprised? I was, but after I read about some of the phytonutrients in this herb, I understood why it could help alleviate allergy symptoms.

Garlic contains quercetin, an excellent immune booster. Quercetin is a plant pigment known as a flavonoid with anti-inflammatory and antioxidant qualities. It's in these capacities that it naturally reduces histamine. This may mean you may be able to reduce your prescription or over-the-counter drugs or eliminate them.

How to Use: The easiest way is to start adding fresh garlic to your favorite dishes. In addition to the spaghetti sauce, you might want to try adding the cloves to soups and stews. Rice and pasta are always good seasoned with garlic.

You might want to bake a clove of garlic. Cut it in half and baste it with olive oil. You'll discover it becomes soft and easy to spread. You can eat them on crackers or bread.

Stinging Nettle leaf

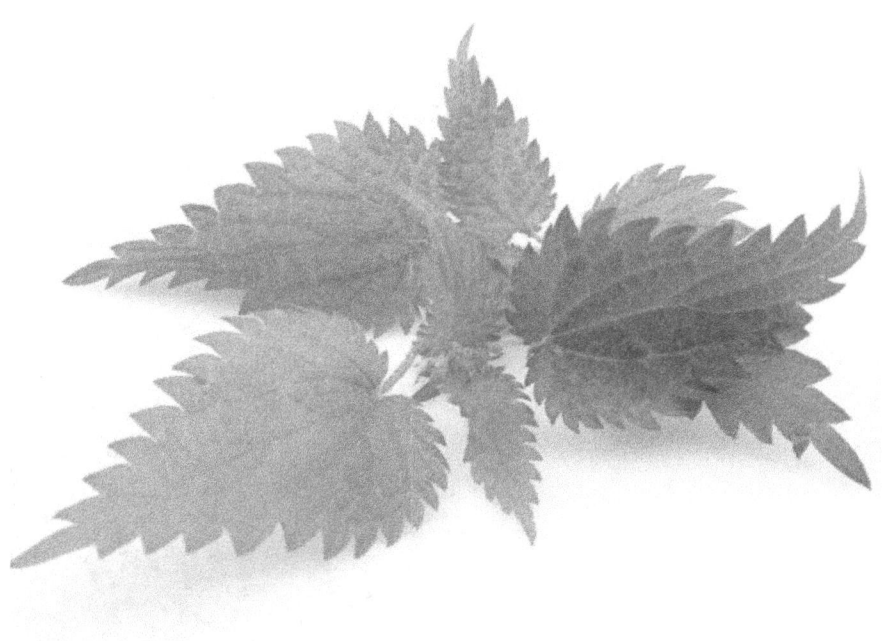

Stinging Nettles is a plant found throughout nearly every region of the United States, and it just may be the remedy to your allergy miseries.

Its anti-inflammatory properties may not only lessen your symptoms, but the latest research shows it may potentially inhibit inflammatory responses.

How to Use: Make a tea or infusion out of the leaves. Use

one teaspoon for each cup of water. Steep this five to 20 minutes. Drink two to three cups a day.

Anxiety

Alfalfa

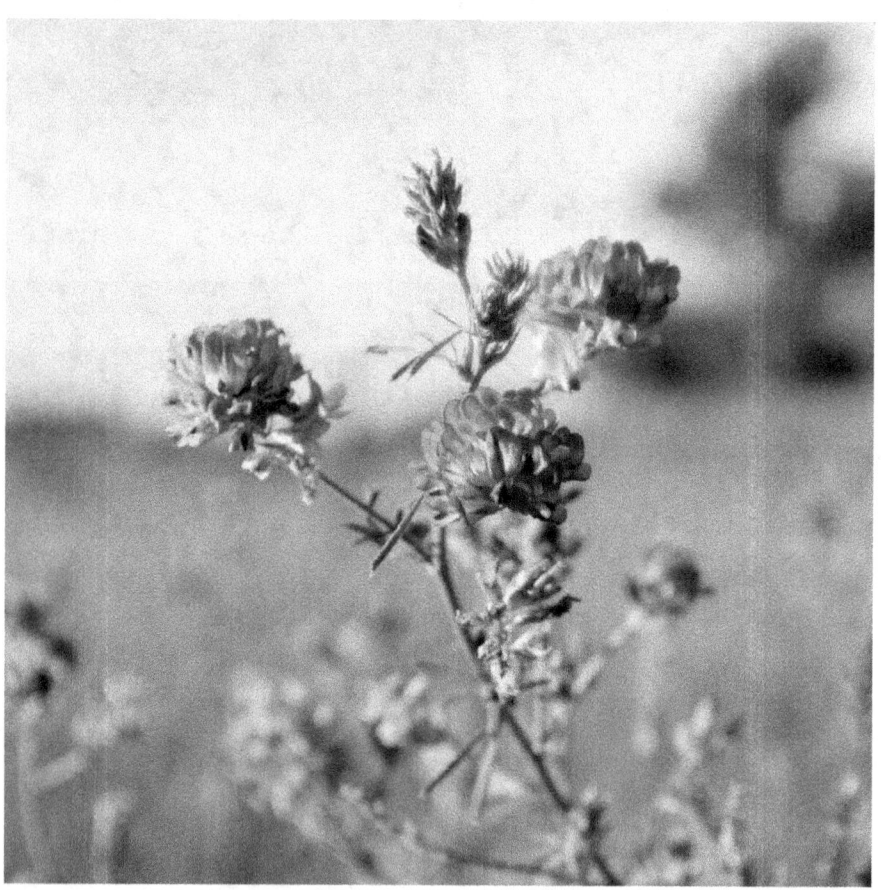

Today, alfalfa is most a cultivated plant, but you can find

it growing wild just about anywhere in North America.

How to Use: Of course, you can add alfalfa sprouts to your salads and other dishes. But you can also make a tea using its dried leaves or crushed seeds. Use one teaspoon of your choice. Allow the leaves to steep for 10 to 15 minutes. The seeds need to boil for up to 30 minutes.

Stinging Nettles

This herb grows naturally throughout the United States.

How to Use: Fresh or dried leaves are best at remedying anxiety and fatigue. They should come from the top of the plant, which is non-flowering. Use them daily as an infusion. Use one teaspoon for each cup of water. Steep this for five to 20 minutes. You may also cook them as you would greens.

Passionflower

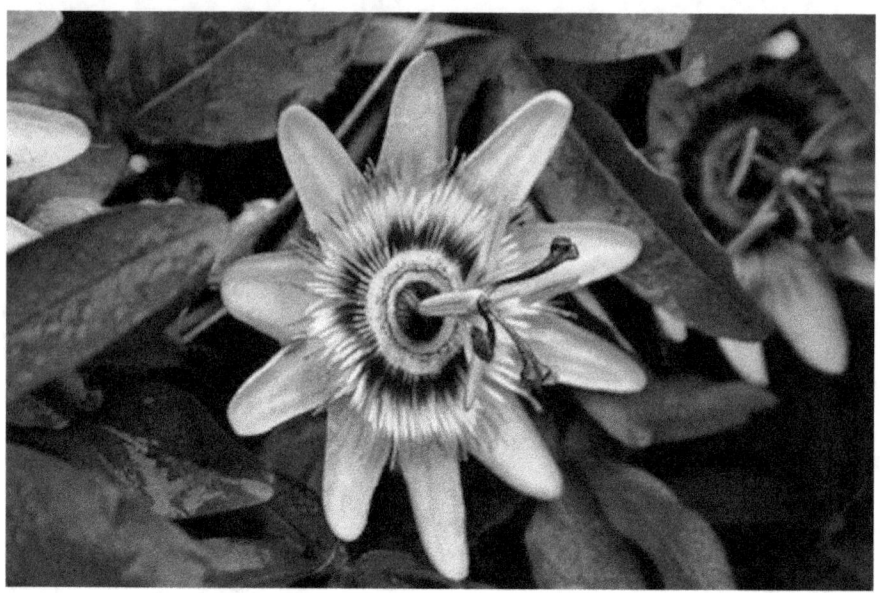

There are about 500 known species of passionflower. This family of plants is also known as Passiflora. Some studies suggest that certain species may have the ability to relieve anxiety. One species is found in Missouri, while others are native to Arizona, Florida, Texas.

How to Use: All you need to do is make a tea from all parts of the dried plant except the root. Use one teaspoon for the dried herb and two teaspoons; if you use fresh, crush them and steep it for six to 10 minutes. Drink this as necessary.

Arthritis

Black Cohosh

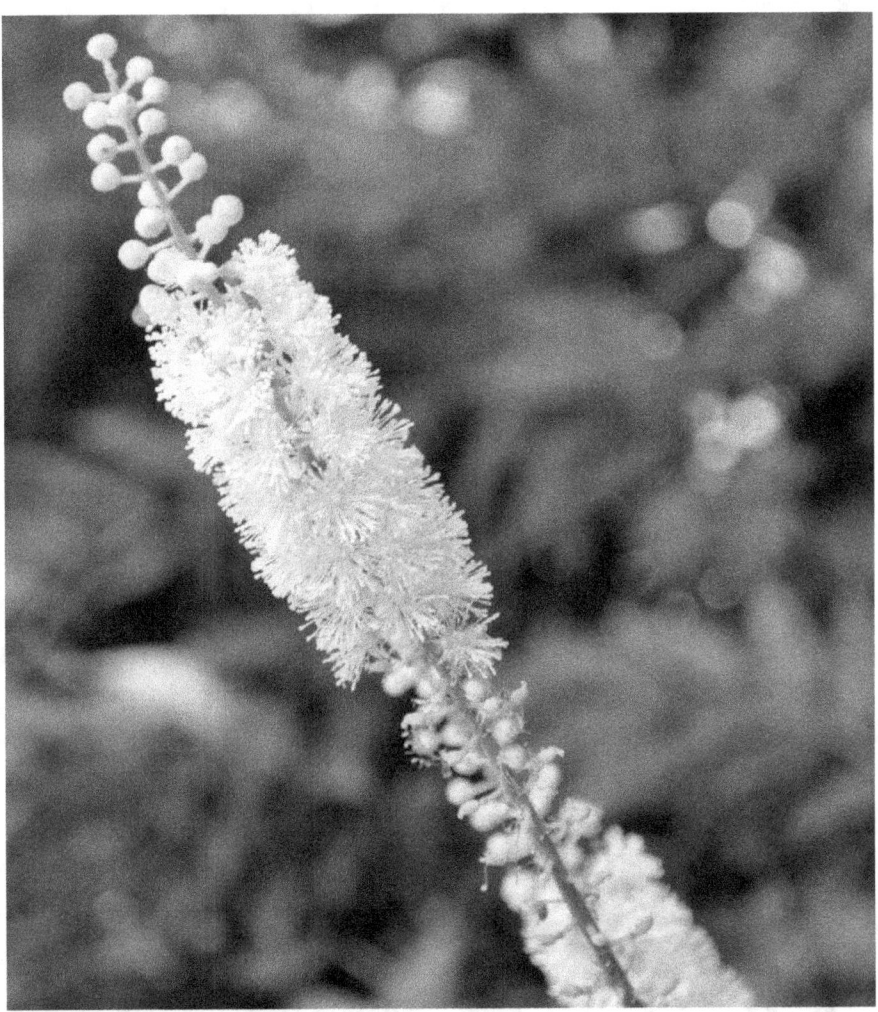

With a botanical name of *Cimicifuga Racemosa*, this plant

grows in eastern North America. It's a member of the buttercup family and also goes by the names of black bugbane, black snakeroot, rattle weed, and fairy candle.

How to Use: To make Black Cohosh tea, use one teaspoon of the dried root for one cup of water. Allow it to steep for about three minutes. If you'd like your tea stronger, you can allow it to steep for up to 15 minutes. You may sweeten naturally if you like.

Boneset

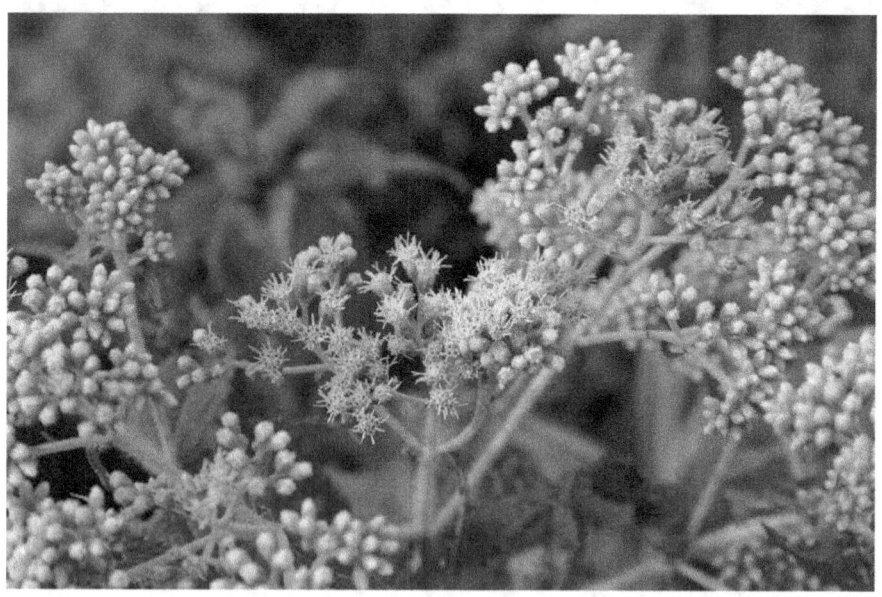

This is another Native American herb with many uses,

one of which is to relieve the pain of arthritis. Its botanical name is *Triosteum perfoliatum*, but you may have heard it called feverwort. It belongs to the honeysuckle family and grows in the eastern regions of North America, especially in the thickets. It also grows from Louisiana as far west as Oklahoma and from Nebraska north to Minnesota.

How to Use: Apply a poultice or balm made from the entire herb to the affected area. Use one tablespoon of the leaves and flowering tops for each cup of water. Steep this for 10 to 15 minutes.

Devil's Claw

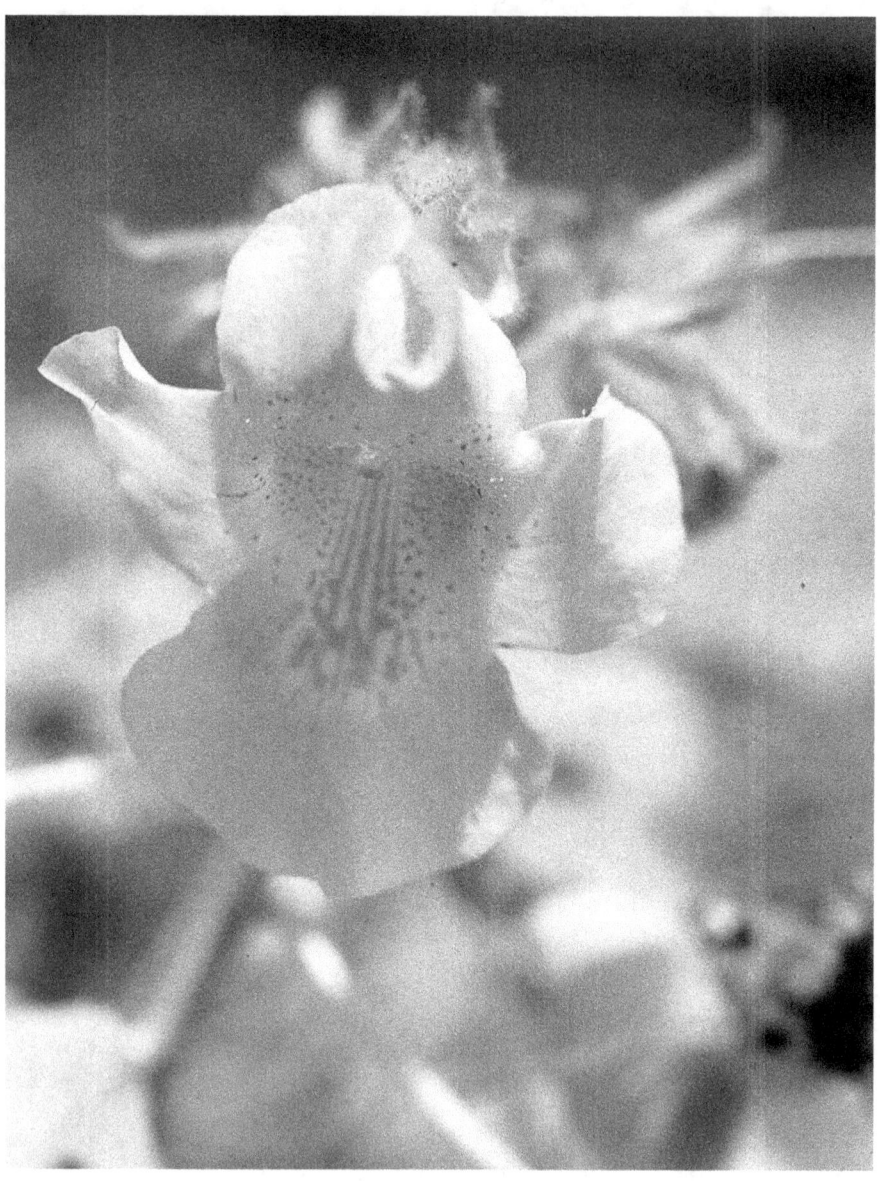

North America is home to several species of this plant

with the botanical name *Proboscidea,* and Native Americans employed it for pain of any type, including arthritis. It grows throughout North America. Other names you may hear it called are Ram's horn, Unicorn plant, or Proboscis Flower.

How to Use: Use the roots and tubers to make a balm or poultice and apply them to the painful joints.

Horsetail

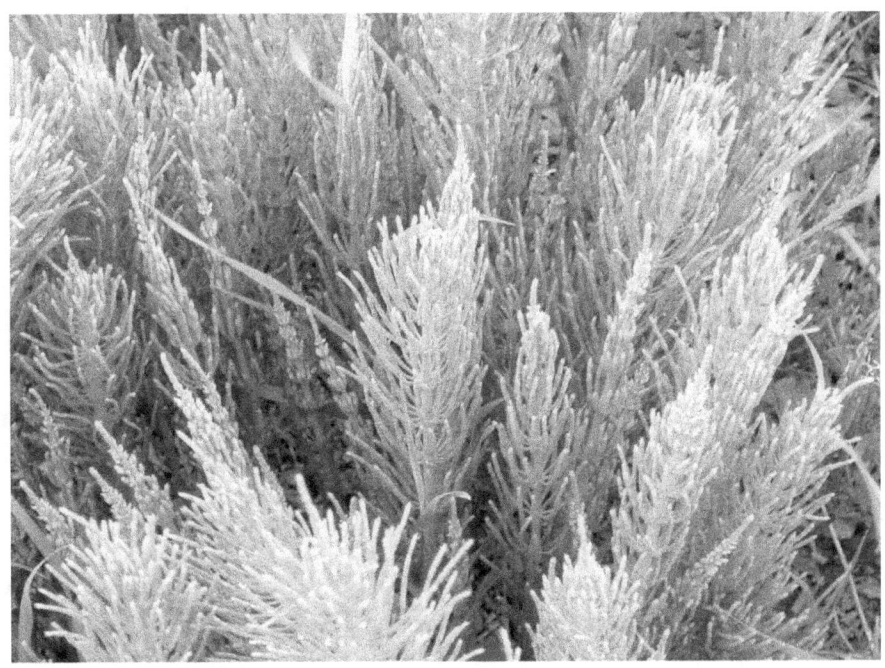

The herb horsetail was one that Native Americans turned to fight the pain associated with arthritis. You may hear it called scouring rush, but know this refers to the same plant with the botanical name *Equisetum*. It grows freely along the stream banks and in the meadows throughout North America.

Science has confirmed its healing ability for arthritis. Horsetail possesses a high silica content, which is essential to bone health.

How to Use: Make a tea or infusion using one large handful of the herb – all parts but the roots—for every two cups of water. Steep this for 15 minutes

Asthma

Apple

Native Americans discovered that by drinking apple water, you could reduce the symptoms of this condition. It may sound simplistic, but today research shows that apples may be the front line of defense of asthma-related breathing problems.

How to Use: Simply slice an apple – any variety will do – and place several slices in a glass of water. Sip this throughout the day. I don't have asthma, and I still drink apple water on occasion. I add a bit of cinnamon to mine. You might want to try that.

Carrot

Native American healers viewed this vegetable as an expectorant, meaning it helped get rid of mucus.

How to Use: The easiest way to gain the healing benefits of carrots is simple to eat more of them, either cooked or raw. You can also make an infusion of the carrots themselves. Use two large carrots, washed but don't peel them. Place them in a pan with five cups of water. Let it steep for five minutes. If you'd like, you can sweeten it or add a bit of ginger to it while it's steeping.

Garlic

This is probably one of the most versatile of the healing herbs, thanks in large part to its anti-inflammatory qualities. Asthma is an inflammatory condition.

Of course, cooking with additional garlic, when possible, is a start at combating asthma.

How to Use: If you're looking for an aggressive approach, you should consider drinking garlic juice. You start with five cloves of crushed fresh garlic, then strain the juice away. Drink this four times a week.

Bad Breath

Parsley

There's a reason why a sprig of parsley is on your plate when you eat out. Yes, it helps to keep your breath fresh. But you don't have to visit your favorite restaurant to get that benefit.

If it isn't already in your herb garden, you can buy the plants just about anywhere. Be careful; you won't need too many since it's an invasive plant and will take over an area if you allow it.

How to Use: Chop parsley leaves finely. Use one teaspoon of dried leaves for each cup of water. Let it steep for five to ten minutes. Or you could just munch on the fresh leaves.

Sage

One of the oldest healing herbs, sage may be an effective remedy against the causes of bad breath. It grows throughout the United States, but it's also a staple in many herb gardens. You can go to any nursery to get some starter plants. *Salvia apiana* is the botanical name for the most common North American species.

How to Use: There are two methods you can try; both involve tea made from the whole leaves. Allow it to steep for about five minutes. You can drink the tea once or twice a day, or you can gargle with it three times a day. Do not use your prepared sage tea if you've had it on hand for more than 24 hours.

Back Pain

St. John's Wort

This versatile plant with the botanical name *Hypericum*

perforatum is a great pain-reliever. You may hear it called Tipton's Weed or Chase-devil. It's considered a weed by many and grows throughout the United States.

How to Use: Use it as an infused oil.

Valerian

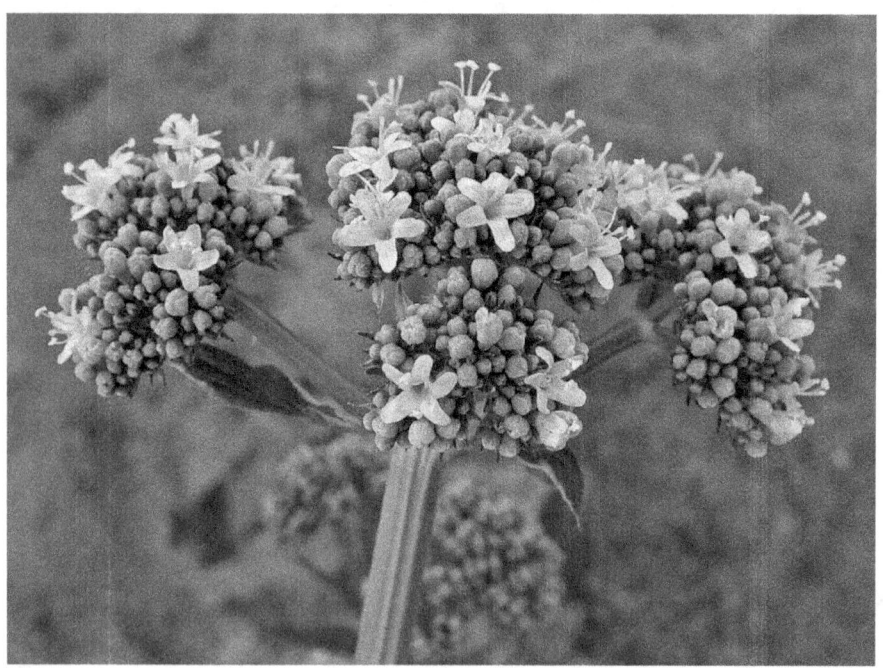

Its botanical name is *Valeriana officinalis* and can be found throughout the northern United States. The herb's amazing pain-relieving properties are due to its natural ability to desensitize your nerves.

How to Use: To take full advantage of this, make tea from the dried roots at a ratio of one teaspoon for each cup brewed. Allow it to steep for about 10 minutes. Drink throughout the day. If you like, you can drink this about 45 minutes before bedtime to help lull you to sleep.

Willow Bark

Considered by herbalists to be the original aspirin, this natural remedy can be used for not only back pain but for general aches and pains. If you're allergic to aspirin, though, you'll want to pass on the remedy.

You can find the willow in temperate regions of North America.

How to Use: Cut dried willow bark or break it into chips, then use approximately one tablespoon of and boil it in water for ten minutes. Remove it from the heat and then allow it to steep for about half an hour.

Burns

Aloe Vera

There are hundreds of species of the aloe plant, and all grow in the warmer climate of North America. It's known as the burn plant and for a good reason. The sap found in the leaves of this succulent plant has remarkable healing properties. Not only does it help to alleviate the burn, but it hastens the healing and reduces scarring.

How to Use: Gently take a leaf from the plant and split it open. Put the sap directly on the burn.

Calendula

The botanical name, *Calendula*, may not be familiar to you, but the common name will be the marigold. It's more than just a pretty face. It just may be the exact thing you need to heal your burn. It works because it possesses antiseptic and anti-inflammatory qualities.

How to Use: This remedy is most effective when you place a compress made from the flowers on the affected area.

Oregon Grape

A native to western North America, this herb was used by the Native Americans to help ease the pain and the healing of burns. Modern scientists have found there's a good reason for the herb's effectiveness. It contains an alkaloid called berberine, which is an antimicrobial.

How to Use: Make that into a poultice from the stems and roots of the herb.

Slippery Elm

Native Americans knew the bark of the slippery elm could heal burns. Botanically called *Ulmus rubra*, this tree grows naturally in eastern North American as well as from southeast North Dakota, eastern Texas, and northern Florida.

How to Use: Make a poultice from the dried bark.

Common Cold

American Ginseng

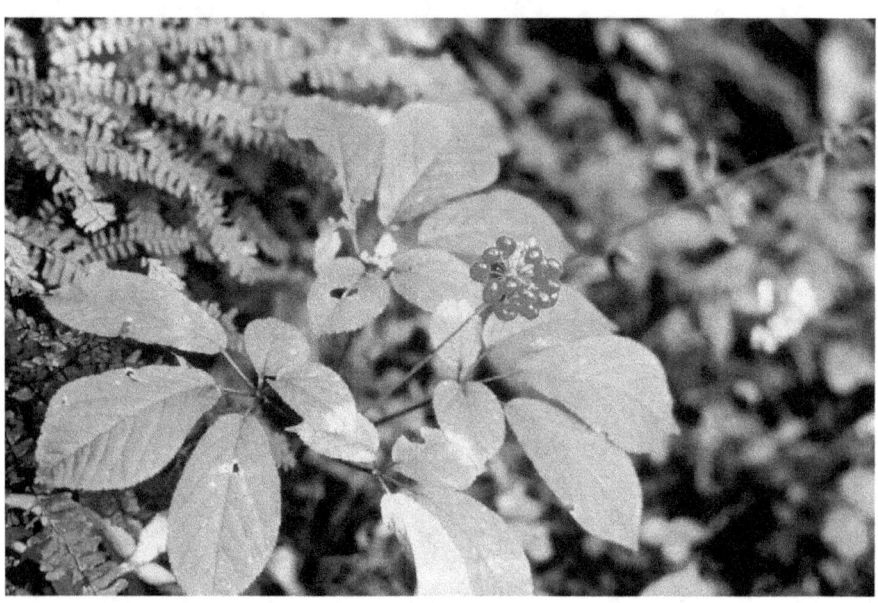

American ginseng, with the botanical name *Panax quinquefolius*, is found in the forests of eastern North America. Native Americans employed this herb long before a European ever set foot on the continent. The Seneca, especially, relied on this to help ease their cold symptoms.

How to Use: One of the most effective methods of preparation is to make a tea from the herb's root using approximately two ounces of root for every eight-ounce cup of water. Steep it for five to ten minutes.

Catnip

We associate catnip with the herb that our feline friends love, but you may want to make it your new friend as well — especially if you're suffering from a cold. Its botanical name is *Nepeta cataria,* and its stems and leaves make an aromatic tea that may just ease the symptoms of a cold.

How to Use: You can make a tea out of this with either dried or fresh leaves and stems. Steep this for five to ten minutes. Drink as you need it.

Echinacea

This is the herb legends are made of. And not only by the Native American herbalists. Today's medical specialists have not only come to appreciate the healing and immune-boosting qualities of Echinacea but have confirmed its effectiveness through rigorous scientific studies. While supplements in all forms are available, you may want to try your hand at using it straight from nature.

A member of the daisy family, echinacea is often referred to as the coneflower or the purple coneflower. This herb won't directly alleviate the symptoms of your cold, but it will do the next best thing: it may noticeably shorten its length.

How to Use: You can make a tea from either the roots, the flower, or its leaves. If you fresh plant parts, use a half cup; if you have the dried herb us a quarter cup. Steep this for up to 15 minutes. You can drink several cups of this a day.

Wild Onion

A cousin of garlic, the wild onion, is also an herbal healing superstar. With more than 600 species and widely found throughout the United States, you'll have little trouble foraging for this plant.

The wild onion has many of the same qualities as garlic. This might not be one of the most enjoyable of remedies, but it's effective.

How to Use: The best way to use it as a tea. Use approximately one half of a large onion for every cup of tea. Allow this to simmer for 30 minutes. If you can't stomach it alone, try adding some honey to taste. This combination will not only aid in alleviating your cold, but it'll also help to ease any cough associated with it.

Willow

The healing power of the original aspirin came from the bark of the willow tree, so it seems intuitive that using it naturally may help ease your cold. And with nearly 400 species of these trees in North America, you should be able to find one not too far from home.

The Natchez tribe use the bark of the red willow to bring down a fever, while the Alabama and Creek Indians made use of it as a bath for the same reason.

Today's herbalists tout the benefits of its bark. What you might not have known is that even the leaves can help you.

How to Use: You can use it as a tincture, using either

fresh or dried bark. It's also effective if taken as a tea. Use one tablespoon of dried leaves to one cup of hot water. Allow it to steep for 15 minutes. Drink at least three cups of this a day. You may have up to six cups if you'd like.

Congestion

Bitterroot

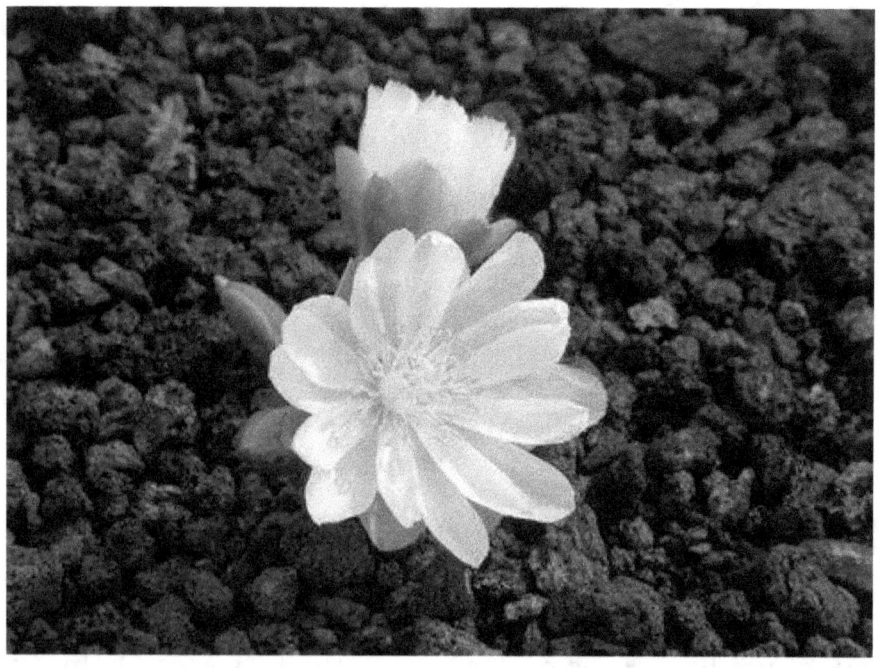

This unassuming flower loomed large in the Native American healing tradition. It bears a single flower, either white or pink, but underneath lies powerful healing roots. With a botanical name of *Lewisia rediviva*, it's found not only on rocky soil but also in grasslands and forests.

How to Use: To make a tea, use about three ounces of the root and allow it to steep for about 15 minutes.

Horsemint

Native Americans made what they called a "sweating tea" from horsemint to treat colds and congestion. Scientifically known as Monarda, horsemint has strong antiseptic properties, thanks to its a substance called thymol. This compound is also found in thyme and provides that herb's distinctive, strong flavor.

You may find it referred to as Oswego tea because it was a popular remedy with that tribe. As a tea, it tastes good. So good, in fact, the English colonists switched to it following the Boston tea party.

Horsemint grows naturally on the east coast from Vermont to Florida and can be found in Minnesota,

Kansas, and New Mexico. This plant loves the sandy prairies, savannas, and sand dunes of the Great Lakes.

How to Use: One teaspoon of the leaves to one cup of water provides the best tasting and more effective remedy for congestion. Allow it to steep for three to five minutes.

Cough

Sage

This herb is versatile and is held to be sacred by many Native Americans. This stems from its purifying effects. Native Americans believe that sage has the ability to cleanse the body and mind of negative energies. To this day, many people, not just Native Americans, use this herb for cleansing purposes.

How to Use: To make sage tea, use two tablespoons of fresh or one tablespoon of the dried herb to one cup of water. Let it simmer for 20 to 30 minutes. You may add honey or lemon or both to taste. You can also gargle with this tea.

Savory

A relative of the rosemary and thyme, savory, can be found in nearly 30 species, all going by the savory name, including Summer savory and Mountain Savory. Its botanical name is *Satureja hortensis*.

How to Use: You can make it as a tea or a poultice for your chest. Use two to four teaspoons to one cup of water. Let it steep for three to five minutes.

Cramps

Chamomile

The same soothing properties that make this herb a great before-bedtime tea also make it an excellent natural remedy for cramps. According to the National Center for Biotechnology Information, this plant has anti-spasmodic properties.

How to Use: You can buy chamomile tea, but for the best results, you'll want to try making the beverage with the fresh herb. To do this, you use three or four tablespoons of the flowers of the herb for one cup of water. Let it steep for three to five minutes.

Cuts

Marshmallow

This isn't the gooey sweet delight you buy at the grocery stores, but there is still a connection. The food was originally made from the sap of the marshmallow plant. Botanists call it *Althaea officinalis*. Today, this herb is more well known for its healing properties, especially it comes to cuts.

How to Use: You can make a poultice out of ground root.

Witch Hazel

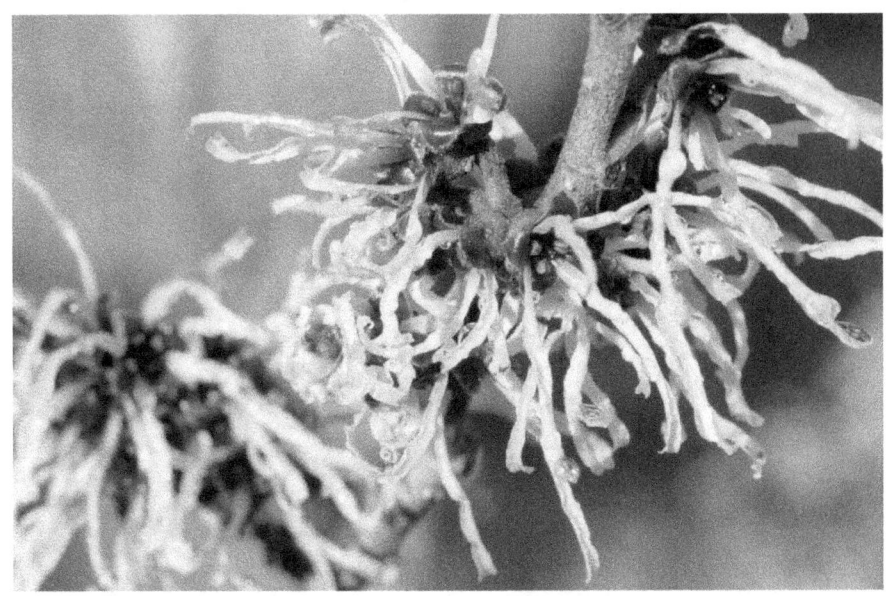

My grandmother always had a bottle of witch hazel in her bathroom medicine cabinet, but it wasn't until I met Grace that I learned it's a plant. This plant is a shrub with the botanical name *Hamamelis virginiana.* You can find it growing as far north as Canada and south in Texas and Florida.

The Native Americans were quick to realize its value as a medicinal herb. The extract of this plant was used to ease help cuts heals as well as treat skin irritations. They also used it to stop bleeding.

And now, instead of reaching for the commercially made variety, you can enjoy the same benefits as the Native Americans.

How to Use: You can make an alcohol-based tincture with the bark and twigs. Use cotton balls, gauze, or a clean washcloth to apply to the affected area.

Yarrow

This plant's ability to heal cuts and wounds is legendary. Its botanical name is *Achillea millefolium*, but you may hear some individuals refer to it as Devil's Nettles. Spanish-speaking cultures call it "plumerillo," meaning "little feather," a reference to the shape of its leaves.

When placed on wounds and cuts, it has the amazing ability to clot the blood and stop the bleeding. That's why you may hear some people refer to the plant as the Nosebleed Plant.

How to Use: Use the leaves of the plant and make a poultice to place.

Depression

Passion Flower

While this plant is found worldwide, there are nine species of it that are native to North America. You find them from Ohio to California and in the Florida Keys. The Native Americans used one of these species, which they called Maypop, extensively and was soon adopted by the colonists. Botanists call it *Passiflora*.

How to Use: Make a tea from the leaves and roots. Steep six to eight minutes.

Warning: Do not use if you are pregnant or breastfeeding.

St. John's Wort

You've probably heard of this herb. It is probably the most common natural remedy for depression. Its botanical name is *Hypericum perforatum*. If you hear people talking about Tipton's Weed or Chase devil, they're referring to St. John's Wort.

St. John's wort is thought to regulate mood by increasing the levels of several chemical messengers in the brain.

How to Use: Make tea with two to three teaspoons of fresh flowers in a cup of water. Let this steep for three to four minutes.

Diabetes

American Ginseng

This plant is an ivy and found in forests from Maine to the Midwest, but it is most plentiful in the Appalachian and Ozarks regions. Its scientific name is *Panax quinquefolius*. The latest research shows that American Ginseng may help to stabilize blood sugar.

How to Use: The root of the plant can be eaten raw, or if you find it a bit hard to chew, steamed. You can also make tea out of the roots. Use two to three teaspoons of the dried herb and allow it to steep for between five and 15 minutes.

Dandelion

So, you doubt that weed on your lawn can help you gain some control over your blood sugar? You shouldn't. Its botanical name is *Taraxacum officinale,* and while you may dismiss it as a weed, but herbalists don't.

To start with it, it's a veritable treasure trove of nutrients, starting with vitamins A, C, D, and B complex. Then add to its nutritional value zinc, iron, and potassium, and you have the makings of a highly effective and useful plant and not just for regulating blood sugar. Herbalists use it a supplemental therapy for kidney disease as well as liver ailments.

How to Use: Dandelion tea can be steeped from any part of the plant, including the leaves, flowers, and roots. Most people use the roots. For a tea made from the flowers, use ten heads or flowers for each cup of tea. Let it steep for up to 20 minutes.

Stevia

You probably know this herb best for its natural

sweetening ability. You may even use it in your coffee or cereal in place of sugar. But did you know it may be able to do even more in your struggle with diabetes?

Stevia is a member of the sunflower family and thrives in subtropical and tropical areas of North America. It's also called Sweetleaf or Sugarleaf.

You're probably thinking if stevia is plentiful in health food and grocery stores, why bother with using fresh. But according to health expert and blogger Halle Cottis, store-bought stevia might not be pure. It might, she suggests, have hidden sugar in it in the form of dextrose.

How to Use: Take the leaves of a stevia plant (if you don't want to forage for it, many nurseries now have it) and dry them. Simply grind them. It's that simple. If you want your stevia in liquid form, take a quarter cup of the powder and mix it with one cup of water. Allow it to sit for 24 hours at room temperature. Then strain the stevia out and use the liquid.

Sumac

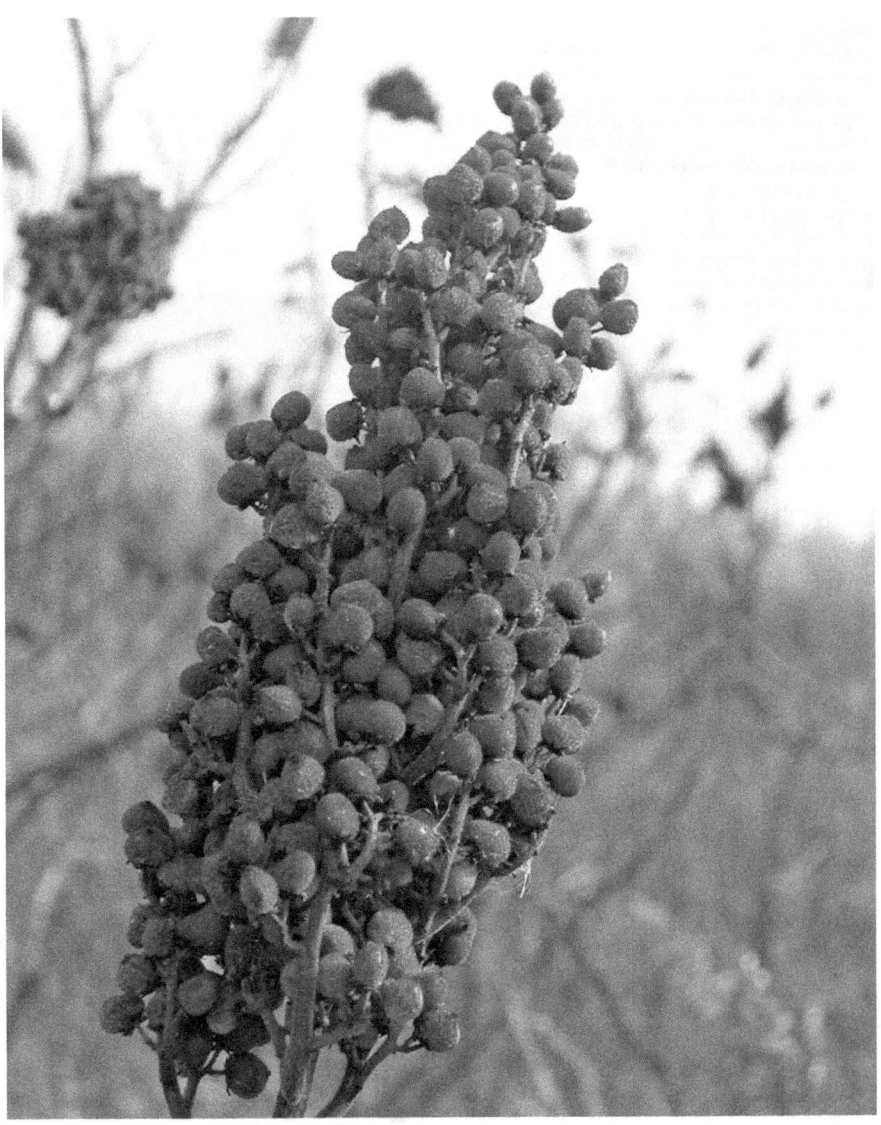

This native North American shrub grows in every mainland state in the U.S. as well as in southern Canada.

It goes by many names, including Dwarf Suma, Mountain Sumac, and Scarlet Sumac, to name just a few. Scientifically, it's called *Rhus*.

This herb was one that Native Americans relied on regularly, not only for medicinal purposes but also for their diet.

How to Use: Make a half-gallon infusion using three to six berry clusters for each half-gallon of water. Allow it to steep between eight and 16 hours.

Wild Carrot

The botanical name for the wild carrot is *Daucus carota*, but you probably know it better as Queen Anne's Lace. You can find what many horticulturists call a weed in nearly every state in the union.

If you're like me, you probably wouldn't aware the below the surface, this lovely lace flower lives a taproot that resembles a carrot and is edible when it's young. But, if you're going to harvest this, be aware that the poison hemlock looks very similar to Queen Anne's Lace, so double and triple check which plant you're harvesting.

The quickest and easiest way to spot the difference between the plants to smell them. If you take a good whiff of Queen Anne's Lace, it smells, not surprisingly, like a carrot. The hemlock, by contrast, smells disgusting.

There is a difference in the appearance of the stem. Queen Anne's is hairy; the hemlock is not.

Of course, the safest way to ensure you choose the right one is by planting Queen Anne's Lace in your garden. Just be aware that it's an invasive plant – that's why it's considered a weed – and may take over much of the space.

The Native American Mohegan tribe used the flowers of this herb as a tea as a treatment for diabetes.

How to Use: Use about five blossoms per cup of tea. When you place the flowers in the water, you'll have to press them down because of their lightweight. Allow it to steep for at least 30 minutes. You can also eat the young root of this plant. When the plant matures, this portion of the plant becomes woody. And if you don't like it raw, try roasting or steaming it.

Diarrhea

American Licorice

This plant's botanical name is *Glycyrrhiza lepidota*, but you may hear people call it wild licorice. It grows just about everywhere in the United States except for a few of the southeastern areas.

The roots of wild licorice are actually quite tasty, and the explorer Meriwether Lewis likened its taste to a sweet potato. Every part of this plant can be used for healing, but the most effective part is the root. Native Americans routinely made an infusion of wild licorice root for diarrhea.

How to Use: You should use approximately one tablespoon of this root for each cup of tea. Allow it to steep for ten or 15 minutes.

Warning: Occasional use of licorice for treating ailments is fine, but if you are using it long-term, it can prompt fluid and electrolyte imbalances. If you're breastfeeding or have heart disease or high blood pressure, you should look for an alternative herbal remedy for diarrhea.

Chokecherry

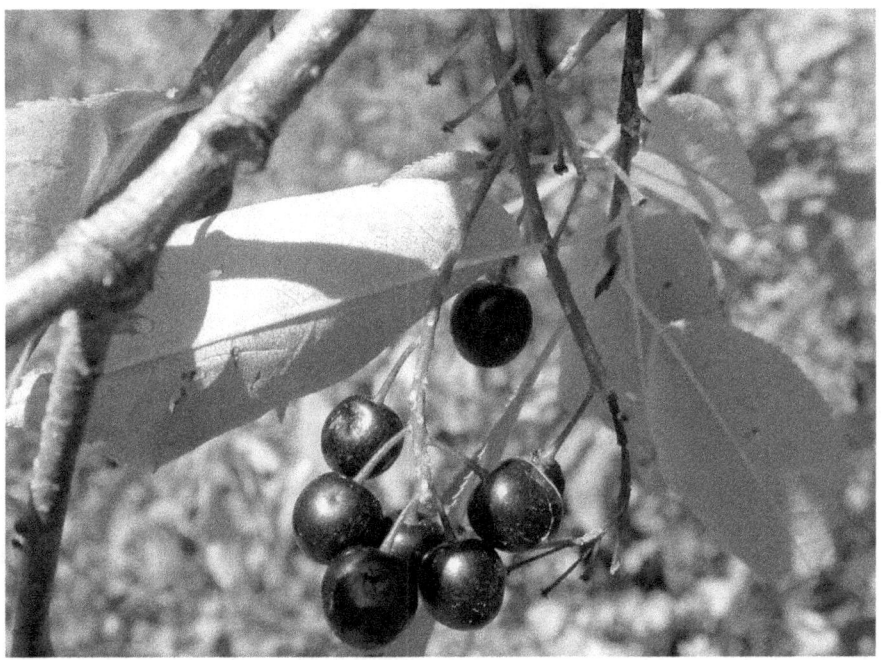

The name doesn't sound like something you want to put into your body, but if you can get past that, you've found yourself a wonderful natural remedy for diarrhea. This herb is also known as Black Chokecherry and Western Chokecherry, and Wild Cherry. It has the scientific name *Prunus virginiana*.

It grows throughout North America and is a popular, effective medicinal tool for tribes like the Delaware, Cree, Iroquois, Chippewa as well as the Mohawk. It is, in fact, considered one of the most important herbs in their herbal tool kit.

How to Use: Use about one tablespoon of the root to a cup of tea. Let this steep three to six minutes.

Geranium

This is another plant familiar to most of us. You might even have some geraniums planted in your garden or around have a border of them around your house. Grace always did. But as you might have guessed, she didn't grow them for their beauty alone, but for their healing powers as well.

If you suffer from diarrhea, this is the flower you want. Its botanical name is *Pelargonium,* and there are plenty of varieties in North America. The Ottawa and Chippewa used the entire plant to make tea to ease the symptoms of this condition.

How to Use: The leaves alone provide plenty of healing. If you choose fresh geranium leaves, use one-quarter cup for each cup of water. If you are using dried, you'll only need two teaspoons. Allow it to steep for about five minutes.

Marshmallow

The marshmallow plant's botanical name is *Althea officinalis* and has been used to treat several different ailments, including diarrhea. It grows in the eastern United States from New York to Florida.

How to Use: You can make a tea using two teaspoons of dried root for every cup of water. Allow it to steep for about five minutes. But don't limit yourself to this method. The flowers and the young leaves are edible. You can boil or fry them or simply add them to your salad.

Digestion

Ginger

The Native Americans used a wide variety of herbs to aid the digestive process. One of the most common was ginger. Wild ginger, known by its scientific name as *Arum canadense,* grows in the forests of eastern North American. It can be found from the great plans east to the Atlantic coast and into the southeastern states.

How to Use: Sipping on ginger tea is probably the easiest way to ease digestive issues. Slice one inch of clean ginger. Allow this to steep for about 15 minutes. If you like, you can add cinnamon or lemon peels.

Burdock

This plant, botanically known as *Arctium lappa*, is a member of the sunflower family. If you hear someone talk about a Cocklebur or a Bardana, they are talking about burdock. The Native Americans used this for many ailments and in a number of interesting ways.

How to Use: Many tribes ate the root to help with digestion. It's the most effective way of reaping its benefits. Wash the roots, then cut one-inch slices. Place these into a bowl to season with olive oil, salt, and pepper. Then spread these roots on a cookie sheet with the cut side down and roast for approximately 15 minutes in a pre-heated oven or until one side is browned, then flip and continuing roasting until the other side is also brown. Believe it or not, this makes a tasty side dish.

But not to worry. If roasted burdock roots aren't to your liking, you can drink its tea. Either fresh or dried burdock will work well. If you have fresh on hand, you'll want about a tablespoon to a cup of water; when you use the dried herb, use between one and two teaspoons. Allow it to steep for about 10 minutes. For best results, drink between two and three cups a day.

Warning: If you are pregnant or nursing, do not use this remedy. Choose one of the other alternatives.

Blackberry

Berries of any kind have been labeled by modern research as superfoods, supplying us with antioxidants and other substances to provide us with robust health. The Native Americans may know this intuitively. They certainly were aware these berries, with the botanical name *Rubus fruticosus*, was a great natural remedy for aiding digestion.

How to Use: They made a tea from the root. And so can you. Just take an ounce of the bark and add it to a pint of water. Allow it to steep for about ten minutes. Drink one or two cups a day.

Dandelion

Who knows this humble plant, nothing more than a weed to us in the United States, could be useful for your digestive issues? My friend Grace knew.

The botanical name of this flower is *Taraxacum officinale*, which is actually a prized healing tool to many herbalists. And with good reason. Today, we know it's a veritable wealth of nutrients, including vitamins A, C, D, as well as the B family. The Mohegans regularly drank dandelion leaf tea as a general health tonic.

The portion of the plant that is most effective for digestive problems is the root, though if you use any of the dandelion, you may find some much-needed relief.

How to Use: Dandelion root tea is best when you roast the roots before making the tea. But don't panic because this fairly easy. Dry the roots, then place them in a pan over medium-high heat until they become golden brown. Then you take about two teaspoons of the roasted root and steep it in water for about 10 minutes. If you don't want to go through the roasting process, you can still get plenty of digestive help by making the tea from the raw roots. You may need to steep them a bit longer.

Dogwood

This plant is as beautiful as it is healing. Its botanical is name *Cornus florida* and grows as far north as Maine and as far south as Florida. It can also be found in several Midwest and western states, including Minnesota, Kansas, and Texas.

You might hear it referred to as American Dogwood or Boxwood, but rest assured, it's the same tree. Native Americans used the bark of the tree as a remedy for digestive issues.

How to Use: Use only the dried bark for the infusion. Fresh bark will only make your stomach and bowels feel worse. Steep one tablespoon in a pint of water for about

30 minutes.

Goldenseal

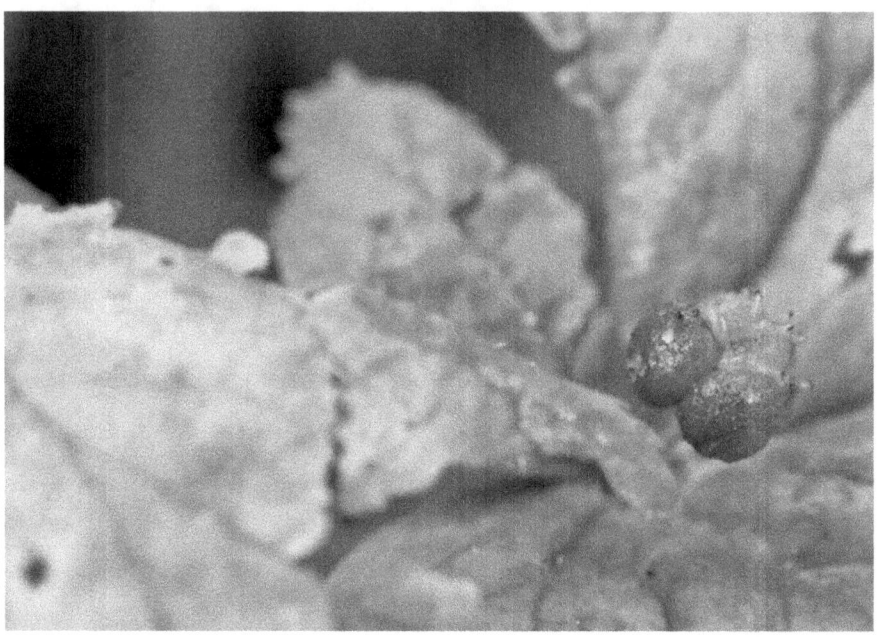

Native Americans knew the healing properties of this
plant long before it was commercially marketed. A
member of the buttercup family, it's also called Orange or
Yellow Root or even Ground Raspberry. Its botanical
name, however, is *Hydrastis canadensis*.

Goldenseal grows mainly in the eastern areas of the
United States, and Native Americans relied on it for more

than just digestive issues. The herb is used even today as an antibiotic and to treat colds and flu.

How to Use: Drink the tea or infusion made from the dried roots or the leaves. Use one teaspoon of the powdered root or leaves to two to three cups of water. Steep for 15 to 20 minutes. If you like, feel free to add a bit of honey or lemon to improve the taste.

Warning: If you're pregnant, do not take goldenseal; find another herbal remedy.

Fatigue

American Ginseng

Let's start with the best. American Ginseng stands head and shoulders above the rest to help you battle that fatigue. The botanical name for this plant is *Panax quinquefolius*, and it has a lot in common with its Asian cousin. If the caffeine in your coffee or tea isn't keeping up with you throughout the day, try American Ginseng. It will give you the energy you need – in a more natural form.

How to Use: You can make a tea or infusion from ginseng root. Use about two ounces of root for every cup of water and drink it throughout the day instead of coffee. Ginseng, however, is a versatile herb, and you can incorporate it into your diet in any number of ways. Lightly steam it to soften the root and eat it as a side dish. Some individuals even like it raw. Or you can add it as a seasoning to soups or stir-fry dishes. Once you put your mind to it and use it routinely, you may be able to kiss your fatigue goodbye.

Rhodiola Rosea

This herb, sometimes shortened to Rhodiola, is another Native American secret herbal remedy for fatigue. You might have heard it called Golden Root, Roseroot, or even Aaron's Rod. All these names refer to the same plant.

Rhodiola Rosea prefers cold weather and can be found in the Rocky Mountains. Not only is this herb an excellent natural treatment for fatigue, but it is also used by the First Americans to boost your mood and help alleviate depression. Not only that, but it also boosts your physical and mental performance.

How to Use: To make Rhodiola Rosea tea, finely cut its roots. Use approximately one teaspoon for two cups. Steep this for about four hours. You may need to adjust the amount of root to find the proper ratio for you.

Fever

American Licorice

This herb also goes by the name of wild licorice and grows throughout the United States except for the southeastern states. With the botanical name of *Glycyrrhiza lepidota*, it has been used not only for fevers but for treating cough and diarrhea. Many Native American tribes used its roots as a tea for bringing down a fever.

How to Use: Finely cut the roots of the herb and use one teaspoon for every cup of tea. Allow it to steep for about 10 minutes. Licorice is naturally sweet, for most likely, you won't want any other sweetener.

Feverfew

A member of the sunflower family, Feverfew's botanical

name is *Tanacetum parthenium*. The benefit of this herb is found right in its name. It comes from Latin and means fever reducer.

How to Use: You can make tea by using a cup of fresh petals or two tablespoons of dried flowers for each cup. Steep for about five minutes.

Feverwort

This herb goes by many names. Wild Coffee, Horse Gentian, Fever-root, and Tinker's Weed. But the most common alternative name you'll find for it is boneset. It carries the scientific name Eupatorium perfoliatum. The Cherokee especially made good use of feverwort tea to reduce a fever.

How to Use: About two teaspoons of the entire herb is needed for each cup of water. Allow it to steep for about 10 minutes.

Willow

Before there was aspirin, the Native Americans used the

bark of the willow tree as a fever reducer. It works so well that its active ingredient, salicin, was the original ingredient in aspirin.

With nearly 400 species of the tree and shrub, it's no wonder the Native Americans relied on this remedy not only as a fever reducer but also for headaches and back pains. The Natchez tribe of the south, for example, used the bark of the red willow. The Alabama and Creek Tribe would take willow root baths as a therapy for a fever. It's abundant and versatile. That makes it a perfect herbal healer.

How to Use: You can use it in tincture form or as a decoction. If you plan on drinking the decoction, then you should be forewarned that it's quite bitter. You may want to add a natural sweetener. Use about one tablespoon of bark chips for each cup of water. Boil it for about 10 minutes and then let it steep another 30 minutes.

Flu

Echinacea

It's no surprise this herb is on the top of the list. Echinacea also goes by the name purple coneflower. It's part of the daisy family and grows in both the prairies and wooden areas. But it's found just about everywhere on the planet. Echinacea is renowned for its healing properties worldwide.

Even today, it's a prized immune booster. But did you realize it has the potential to shorten the length of your illness? Native Americans would chew the roots. If that doesn't sound very appetizing to you, you'll be relieved to know they also made teas out of the leaves. That works just as well.

How to Use: To prepare this remedy as to a tea, you can use either the dried or fresh leaves. If you choose the fresh variety, you'll need twice the amount of dried. That would be a half cup of fresh leaves or a quarter cup of dried echinacea leaves for a cup of tea. Allow it to steep for about 15 minutes. Alone the herb isn't that appealing, so you may want to add honey or another sweetener to it.

Goldenrod

The Native Americans used this plant, with the botanical name *Solidago canadensis* or *Solidago virgaurea,* for centuries. They used it primarily to heal wounds, but it has so many more uses, including fighting the flu.

How to Use: Use two tablespoons of the fresh flowers for each cup of tea you brew. Allow it to steep for about 15 minutes. If you want, you may sweeten it with honey. If you want, you can make a tincture of goldenrod.

Native Hemlock

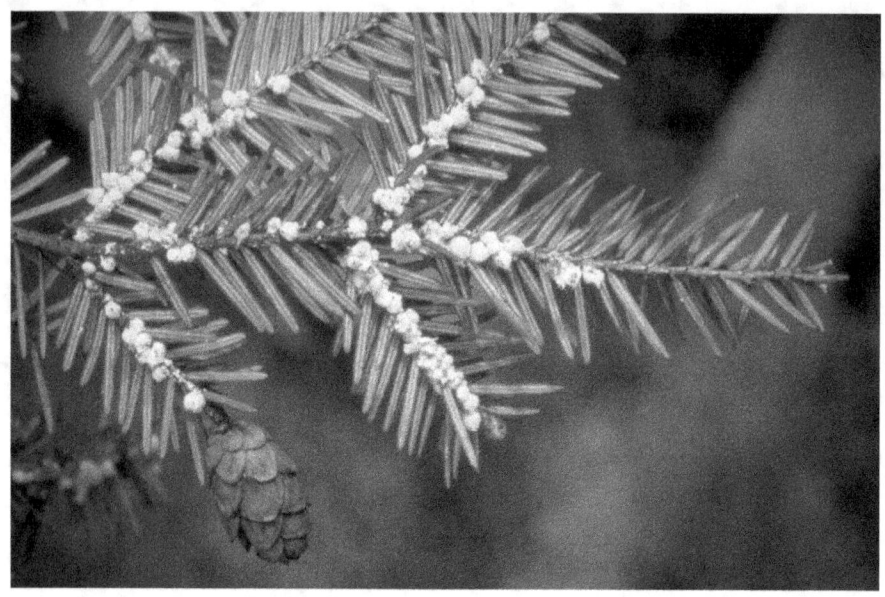

I know what your first thought is. You really don't expect me to take the same herb that killed Socrates? No, I don't. Not in a million years. Native hemlock, known to botanists as *Tsuga*, is a member of the pine family. This species is not in the least bit poisonous.

The Native Americans made good use of Native Hemlock. They applied the pitch in poultice form or as a salve for a diverse number of ailments from colds to sunburn. The Menominee and the Forest Potawatomi utilized the tree's inner bark and its twigs for tea to relieve the flu and the common cold.

How to Use: Don't worry; you won't have to dig for the inner bark of Native Hemlock to make your tea. There's an easier way. You can make a tea that works just as well from the needles of the hemlock. Get half of a handful of the needles and cut them so they are about an inch long, and pour boiling water over it. Allow it to steep for about ten minutes.

Osha

I had never heard of Osha before I met Grace, but she told me it's a member of the celery family. Botanists call it *Ligusticum porteri*, but others often call it Osha Root Bear Root or Bear medicine. It also goes by the name of Colorado Cough Root, which gives you a good indication of how the Native Americans used it.

It grows in the mountainous woodlands throughout the southwest. While every part of Osha can be used for healing, it's the taproot that is the most beneficial. This plant was so highly prized that Native Americans traded it. Tribes located where the plant wasn't indigenous were able to use the herb for their healing and other ceremonies.

Native American culture tells us Osha tea has warming properties. They used it not only for the flu but for colds and to stimulate circulation.

How to Use: Take a handful of the dried root to about three cups of water. Allow this to simmer for at least a half-hour and up to six hours. The tea will contain a translucent, grey-brown tint when it's at its most beneficial. This is one herbal tea that you'll find tastes good. It has a peppery celery taste to it, almost like anise. By the way, while it's simmering, your home will smell as wonderful as the tea tastes.

Gout

Goldenrod

Goldenrod gets a bad rap as being the cause of your allergies. Rest assured your squabble is with ragweed. You can take full advantage of this plant to help ease the pain of your gout without experiencing problems. Its botanical name is *Solidago canadensis* or *Solidago virgaurea.*

How to Use: The best use of goldenrod for the treatment of gout is by drinking its tea. You'll need about two tablespoons of fresh flowers for every cup of tea. Allow it to steep for about 15 to 20 minutes.

Juniper

Another herb that may help the pain of inflammation of gout is the Juniper, or as it's known by botanists, *Juniperus communis*. It's an evergreen shrub that grows in the mountains. The female trees produce cones with small round bluish-black berries. When they ripen, they can be eaten raw or used in teas.

How to Use: Use one tablespoon of the crushed berries for one cup of water. Steep for approximately 10 minutes. If you'd like, you can sweeten it to taste with honey.

Slippery Elm

Slippery Elm's botanical name is *Ulmus rubra,* and it's

native to a scattering of regions in North America. It grows in eastern North America and southeast North Dakota. You can find it as south as the northern tip of Florida as well as in parts of eastern Texas.

Native Americans used it to treat gout and other arthritic conditions, as well as bronchitis and cough.

How to Use: The effective part of the tree is the inner bark. You have two ways of using this valuable herb. First, you can make tea out of the powdered elm bark. Use one tablespoon for every cup. Steep for three to five minutes. If you like, you can add honey or cinnamon. Or you can apply a poultice to the affected area.

Wild Rose

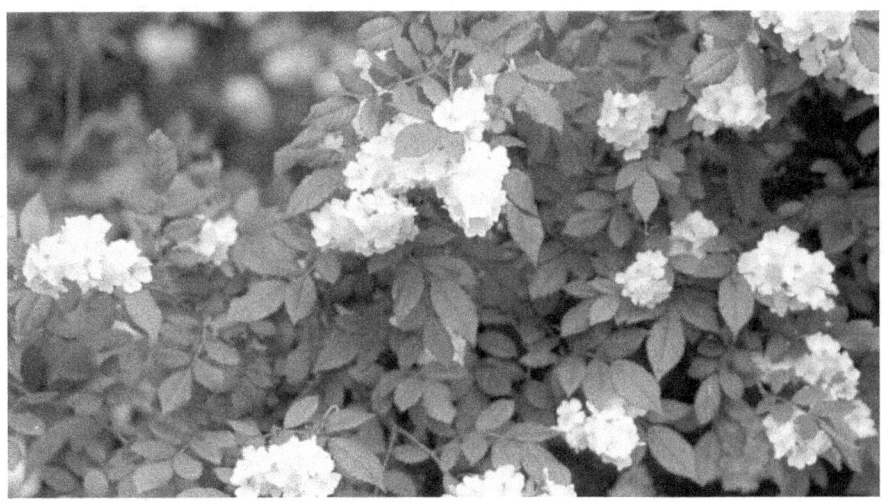

Wild Rose, or *Rosa multiflora*, has been used for healing for thousands of years. You may know it better as Sweetbriar, Briar Rose, Brier Hip, or Dogberry. It's native to wooded areas as well as open areas. In fact, the wild rose is found just about everywhere in North America.

While the Native Americans not only used it to treat the pain of gout and other arthritic conditions, but they employed this herb for digestive issues, stress as well as for the common cold.

How to Use: Treat yourself to a cup or two of tea from its

petals for relief. If you use fresh petals, use one-quarter cup to one cup of tea. Allow it to steep for at least 10 minutes. For tea made from the dried leaves, you only need one to two teaspoons.

Headache

Black Cohosh

With a botanical name of *Cimicifuga racemosa*, this plant grows in eastern North America. It's a member of the buttercup family and also goes by the names of black bugbane, black snakeroot, rattle weed, and fairy candle. The Oklahoma Delaware, as well as the Winnebago and Dakota tribes, all employed this valuable herb as a remedy for a headache.

How to Use: To make Black Cohosh tea, use one teaspoon of the dried root for one cup of water. Allow it to steep from three to 15 minutes, depending on the strength. You may sweeten naturally if you like.

Broom Snakeweed

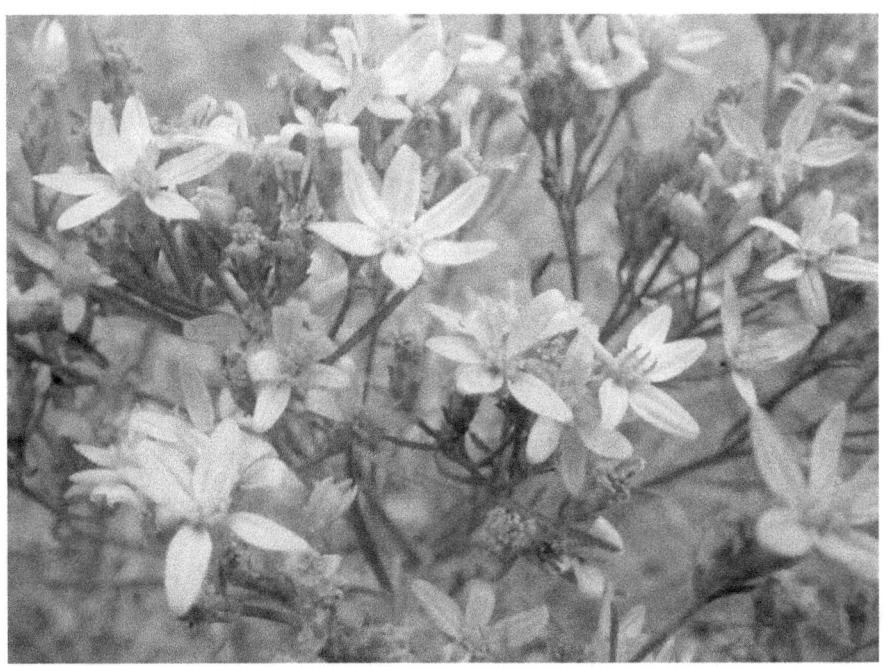

Botanists call it *Gutierrezia sarothrae*; others simply call it snakeweed. However, you identify it one thing is sure: it's a great natural remedy for a headache. The Navajo knew this too. This was their go-to healing herb for that affliction.

But Broom Snakeweed has some other talents as well. The Sioux employed this herb for coughs and colds, and interestingly enough, vertigo. The Blackfoot inhaled the steam of the boiled roots for respiratory ailments.

How to Use: If you want to use the traditional Navajo therapy (and really, who wouldn't), then you need to burn the herb and rub the ashes on your head. If you are not quite so adventurous, you may want to make a strong tea out of the herb and use it as a poultice.

Cardinal Flower

Its botanical name is *Lobelia cardinalis*. You can recognize this instantly because of its bright red flowers. It grows in the eastern and southwestern regions of the United States.

Native Americans found this an excellent remedy for headaches as well as colds and cramps.

How to Use: Use the roots of this flower as a poultice and place it in the area your head hurts.

Feverfew

This herb, a member of the sunflower family, is legendary in herbal healing literature. Its botanical name is *Tanacetum parthenium*. In addition to relieving headaches, especially migraines, Feverfew is an excellent remedy for treating fevers, arthritis, and digestive issues.

How to Use: To bet the best relief, you can drink it as a tea. Simply use one tablespoon of fresh flowers for each cup of water. Steep it a minimum of 30 minutes and a maximum of 60. Drink one or two cups a day.

Peppermint

This is another herb with a fine healing pedigree. With the botanical name of *Mentha Piperita*, it's actually a hybrid of the water mint and spearmint. It grows just about everywhere in North America and is especially found near streams and other wet places.

Peppermint has a natural numbing effect, which makes it a perfect remedy for a headache. It is also used by some people for anxiety and depression.

How to Use: Use four or five spears of the mint for two cups of water and let it steep for about five minutes. You can make peppermint into a poultice and place it on the area or your head that hurts.

Warning: Don't give peppermint to an infant or small child. It can cause severe breathing problems.

Heart and Circulatory Issues

Hawthorn

This is the herb for heart issues. The Native Americans used it not only to treat cardiovascular problems but also to prevent them. This plant grows in the temperate areas of North America.

To show you its immense healing ability, one of the first heart medications, Digitalis, was made from this herb. Numerous studies demonstrate its amazing ability to help the heart.

Don't expect to use it for a day or even a month and see improvement in your heart condition. Hawthorn is definitely classified as a long-term remedy. You'll need to use this plant for at least several months – and may several years – to feel its full benefits.

How to Use: To make hawthorn tea, steep one heaping

teaspoon of the combination of the flowers and leaves (or either one singly) and let it steep for 15 to 30 minutes. Drink no more than three cups daily.

To make a tincture of hawthorn, place the leaf and flower in a glass jar and cover it with alcohol. Allow it to sit for a minimum of two weeks. In place of the leaf and flower, you can use either fresh or dried berries. Take 30 to 40 drops three to four times a day.

Indian Hemp

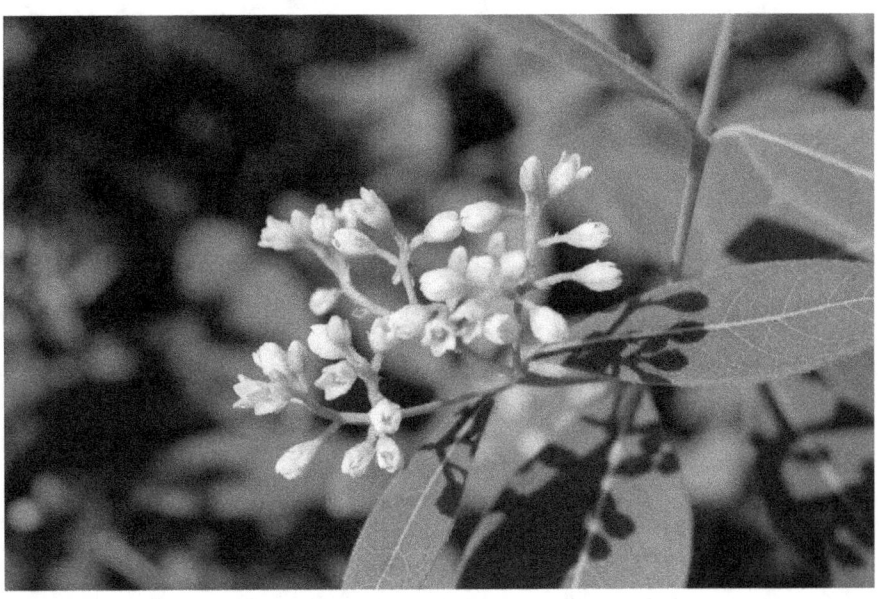

The botanical name for this plant is *Apocynum*

cannabinum and also goes by American hemp, Dogbane, Amy Root, Hemp Dogbane Wild Cotton, or Rheumatism Root. And yes, it is a variety of marijuana. Indian Hemp grows throughout much of North American and likes gravelly or sandy soil. It can be found near streams. It is a much sought-after natural heart remedy.

How to Use: Take one teaspoon of dry hemp leaves for each cup of water. Hemp is not water-soluble, so it's best to drink this tea with a splash of milk.

Prickly Pear Cactus

There's something unique about the prickly pear cactus. It is not only classified as a vegetable but also as fruit and even a flower. As you might expect, it is native to the southwestern United States. With the botanical name of *Opuntia engelmannii*, it's also known as Cow's Tongue Cactus, Desert Prickly Pear, and Texas Prickly Pear.

The Native Americans used this cactus as a food source as well as a healing herb. The younger pads of the plant were eaten, and the older ones were used as a poultice. They also made teas from the plant.

How to Use: To make a cactus tea, take 1 ½ teaspoons of the berries to one cup of water. Steep for four minutes.

Perhaps the best way to make use of the healing powers of the prickly pear cactus is to incorporate it into your diet. You can include the leaves in your smoothies or make a juice out of them. There are also several recipes for prickly pear cactus. The uses of this plant are limited only by your imagination.

Wild Garlic

There are many species of this herb in North America, but the most plentiful is the allium canadense. It goes by many names, including Canadian garlic, meadow garlic, and even Canada onion. It grows in the eastern regions of North America and from Texas to Florida. You may also be able to find it in some western states, especially Montana.

The Native Americans used this plant for a variety of ailments in addition to heart disease. They employed it as a remedy for indigestion, asthma, and even loss of appetite. And there is a good reason so many people today use it for their heart. Garlic possesses a chemical called allicin, which is a type of antioxidant. And they contain one more heart-healthy antioxidant: quercetin. And if you get this important nutrient through garlic, your body absorbs it easier.

How to Use: Are you ready to reap all the health benefits wild garlic has to offer? You might want to start by drinking garlic tea. I know it doesn't sound very appetizing, but feel free to sweeten it with a little honey or add ginger to improve the taste. Steep a clove of minced or chopped garlic in a cup of water. And allow it to steep for about five minutes. You can also use it as an infused oil.

Heartburn

Dandelion

This pesky weed that seems to be everywhere may just be your ticket to eliminating your heartburn. Why? It's rich in vitamins A, C, and D, as well as the B family. But it also has an abundance of minerals for a plant so small: iron, potassium, and zinc.

The Pillager Ojibwas drank the roots of the plant as a heartburn remedy, while the Mohegan drank its leaves as an all-purpose health tonic.

How to Use: If you choose to use the roots with which to prepare your decoction, use two tablespoons of the root coarsely chopped for one cup. Allow this to steep for about 40 minutes.

If you use the leaves, you'll want to use about two teaspoons of the dried and crushed leaves for one cup of tea. Allow this to sit between five and 10 minutes, depending on the strength you desire. You can drink this hot or cold.

Osha

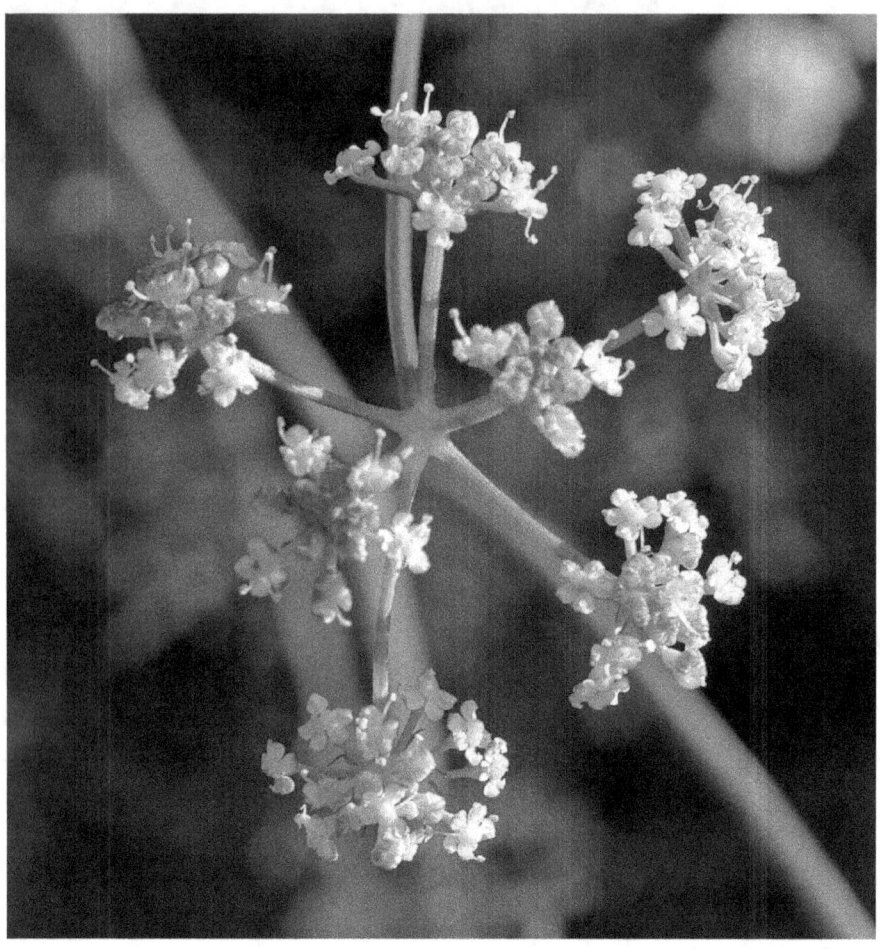

You may hear this herb called Porter's Licorice Root,
Osha Root, or Bear Root. Botanists refer to it as
Ligusticum porteri. It's a cousin to celery. Grown in the
mountains and woodlands of southwest North America, it
was prized by Native Americans as a valuable, effective

herbal remedy. While It may have been found only in a limited region, Osha's healing powers were known by all tribes. Native Americans used it as trade. This allowed others to not only use it for healing but employ it for other ceremonies as well.

Every part of this plant is used for healing purposes, but it's the taproot that is the most valuable and beneficial. The roots were used in teas and poultices.

How to Use: With a handful of the dried roots, you can make three cups of tea. Simmer this for at least half an hour. Actually, if you can wait up to six hours, you'll get the most benefit and the best taste from the drink.

The tea will look translucent and have a grey-brown tint to it. That's when you know you've achieved the perfect strength. It will remind you of anise, with a peppery celery taste. This tea will do more than relieve your heartburn. The added bonus is that it makes your home smell wonderful.

Stevia

Like me, you might already use stevia as a natural sugar substitute. But Grace told me about its near-magical properties of relieving heartburn.

A member of the sunflower family, you can find nearly 240 types of stevia in North America. It grows in the subtropical and tropical regions of the continent. You can find it in the northwest all the way to South America.

How to Use: You don't want to make a tea out of stevia alone, but you can use the fresh leaves (harvest from the top, and the plant will grow bushier). Depending on your taste, you can use up to four leaves in a regular herbal tea. You can also put the leaves in a food processor and grind them to use in place of sugar for your baking needs.

White Pine

Botanists call it *Pinus strobus*, but you may hear it referred to as Deal Pine and Soft Pine. This tree grows from Newfoundland down to Georgia mountains on the east coast as well as in central Iowa and northern Illinois.

Native Americans have long used its inner bark, young shoots, and twigs, as well as the pitch and needles for everything from the common cold to pneumonia to heartburn and arthritis.

How to Use: The easiest way to make use of the tree as a heartburn remedy is with a tea of pine needles. Don't knock it till you try it. Grace made this for me once and didn't tell me what she made it with. You'll like it – especially if it can ease that heartburn.

The recipe is simple. You'll want to take a large handful of young pine needles. If they are any brown ends, break them off. Don't use them. Chop the green ones into pieces of about half an inch. Place them in a container of glass, ceramic or stainless steel. Pour two cups of boiling water over them and allow them to steep for about five minutes. When I first made my own, I was surprised at how short a time they need in the water. When the tea is ready, it will have a pale green look to it and, as you might have already guessed, a smell of pine. And it tastes better than it has any right to. If you like, you can add some lemon.

Hypertension (High Blood Pressure)

Hawthorn

If you had to select one herb for any type of heart issue, including hypertension, you might want to choose hawthorn. It's the super herb for these issues.

Found in the temperate areas of North America, mostly east of the Rocky Mountains, hawthorn is also known by its botanical name of *Crataegus*. You may also hear it referred to as quickthorn, thornapple, or May-tree.

Keep in mind that herbs are long-term remedies, and this is especially true of hawthorn. It may take up to several months or more for you to reap its benefits. But you'll discover that when it concerns this herb, patience is, indeed, a virtue.

How to Use: To make hawthorn tea, steep one heaping teaspoon of a combination of the flowers and leaves (or either one singly) and allow it to steep for 15 to 30 minutes. Drink no more than three cups daily.

You can also make a tincture using both the leaves and flowers. Many herbalists suggest taking 30 to 40 drops three to four times a day.

Hummingbird Blossom

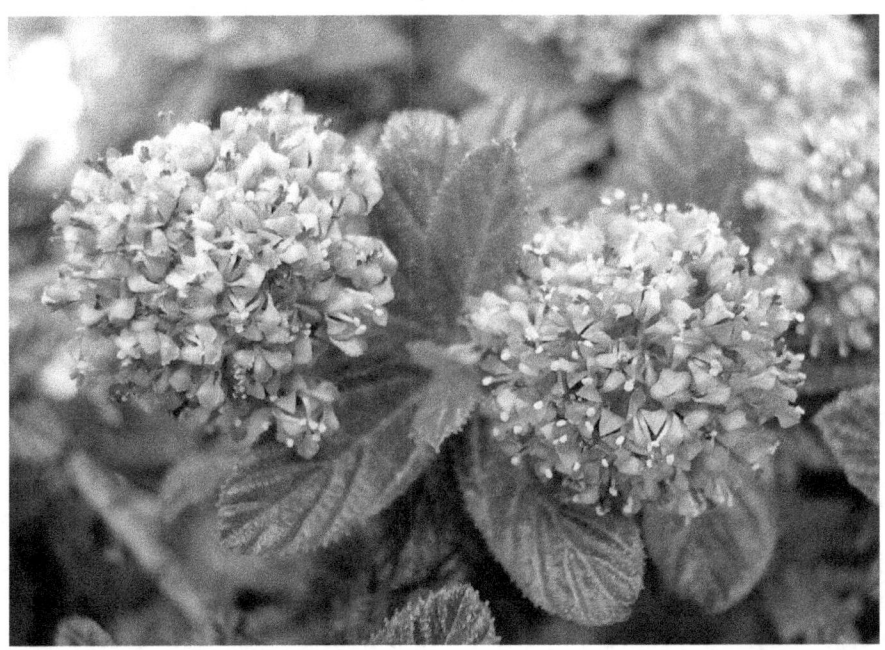

Native Americans used this versatile herb to treat many conditions, including high blood pressure. Found in the western states of Oregon and California, its botanical name is *Ceanothus cuneatus* and is also commonly called buck brush.

How to Use: Use approximately two teaspoons of the ground root for each cup of water. Let this steep for approximately five minutes. Feel free to adjust the amount of herb, depending on your taste.

Parsley

The herb parsley, botanical known as *Petroselinum crispum*, was used by Native Americans for a number of ailments, including those of the heart. Perhaps that's one of the reasons Grace always had it growing just about everywhere – by the side of her house along with her flowers as well as her vegetable garden.

Warning: If you're wildcrafting, be extra careful that you're actually harvesting parsley. There are three other herbs that look very similar, but they're poisonous: Dog poison or fool's parsley and two species of poison hemlock.

Parsley is easy to grow. Sometimes too easy. If you decide to grow an herb garden, you may find this plant reproduces fast and overcrowds your other herbs.

How to Use: There's an easy way to get your parsley

regularly to help remedy your high blood pressure. You put a pinch of the herb with the fresh juice of one lemon and a glass of water in the juicer. It's best to drink this on an empty stomach. Many individuals use this in the morning, wait 15 minutes and then eat their normal breakfast. You can use this for 15 days. Abstain from it for five days and then start another 15-day regimen.

Parsley also makes a wonderful tea. You can use either fresh or dried leaves. You'll need one-quarter cup of fresh and two teaspoons of dried for each cup.

If you prefer, you can make a decoction from the roots of this herb. In this case, you'll use one to two tablespoons of the root for each cup of tea.

Wait. There's one more way you can make parsley tea, and that's from its seed. For each cup you make, use two teaspoons of seeds. Steep this for about five minutes.

Stevia

It may come as a surprise that the same natural sweetener you use in your coffee may also help lower your blood pressure. A member of the sunflower family, stevia grows naturally in the subtropical regions of North America. It's also known as sweet leaf and sugar leaf.

How to Use: Turn to stevia as a natural sweetener every chance you get, especially in herbal teas. You may also garnish your meals with fresh leaves.

Immune System

Echinacea

This herb also called the purple coneflower, is the most potent choice for a better immune system. It's native to the eastern and central regions of North America and can be found not only on the dry prairies but also in open wooded areas. The Plains tribe used it, and the Cheyenne prized it enough to incorporate it in their traditional Sun Dance ceremonies.

How to Use: A cup (or two) of echinacea tea will go a long way in enhancing your immune system. If you use fresh leaves, use half a cup to one cup of water. For dried leaves, the ratio is a quarter cup of leaves to one cup of water. Steep for up to 15 minutes.

Prickly Pear Cactus

This plant, which is classified as a fruit, a vegetable well as a flower, goes by the botanical name of *Opuntia engelmannii*, is another immune-enhancing herb. It grows in the southwestern United States as well as in northern Mexico. You may hear it referred to as Cow's Tongue Cactus or Desert Prickly Pear.

Prickly Pear Cactus served not only as a healing herb but a part of the Native American diet as well. The young pads were eaten; the older pads were made into poultices. The cactus's berries were made into tea.

How to Use: Make a tea of its berries. Use a ratio of 1 ½ teaspoons of the berries to one cup of water. Steep for about five minutes. You can also add the leaves to your morning smoothies or make prickly pear cactus juice.

Infection

Cattail

With a scientific name of *Typha* and approximately 11 species, Cattail grows in the wetlands of the United States. You may also have heard it called Corndog Grass or Bullrush.

But what you might not have heard of its amazing ability to aid in ridding your body of an infection. But the cattail is remarkable for another reason: nearly every part of it is edible.

How to Use: The roots can be cooked and eaten. To prepare the cattail root, clean them and snip off the smaller branching roots, leaving you with the main large one. The root can be boiled, baked, or grilled until its tender.

The spike at the top of the tail is called the pollen, and it's a rich source of protein. Boil this between 10 and 12 minutes before you enjoy its benefits.

The small shoots and stubs found at the base of the plant are called corms and are also edible. Remove and peel them, and you'll discover their tender centers. You can eat these raw or cooked to your preference.

And then there are the shoots. They're also called spikes or stalks. Rinse these and soak them in vinegar to remove any bacteria. You can fry these in butter or olive oil or eat them raw.

Echinacea

Add healing an infection to the list this superstar herb can do. A member of the daisy family, Echinacea is best known for its amazing ability to boost your immune system, which may contribute to the herb's ability to heal infections.

It also goes by the name purple coneflower and grows in the eastern and central regions of the United States.

How to Use: Use the leaves of this plant to make a healing tea. When you use fresh leaves, place a half cup of leaves in one cup of water; for dried leaves, use only a quarter cup. Allow this to steep for up to 15 minutes.

Goldenseal

This versatile herb performs many tasks in maintaining your wellbeing, not the least of which is helping clear infections. Goldenseal belongs to the buttercup family and grows in eastern North America. Botanists call it *Hydrastis canadensis*, but you may hear others call it Ground Raspberry or Orange Root.

How to Use: This herb is most efficient as a tea. Use one teaspoon of either the root in powdered form or the leaves to two or three cups of water. Steep this for three to six minutes. You may want to add either honey or lemon for a better-tasting drink.

Warning: Do not take goldenseal if you are pregnant; use an alternative remedy.

Wild Rose

This plant is legendary for its medicinal qualities, and with good reason; its fruit is an abundant source of vitamin C. While it grows through the wooded areas throughout North America, it's also found in open fields.

How to Use: You can make tea or an infusion from the flowers' petals. If you use fresh leaves, you'll need a ratio of a quarter cup of leaves to one cup of water. When you use dried leaves, you only need one or two teaspoons. Let this steep, covered, for up to 15 minutes.

Inflammation

American Ginseng

If you've used and enjoyed the benefits of Asian Ginseng, then you'll love its American cousin. With a botanical name of *Panax quinquefolius*, this herb's abilities extend to reducing inflammation.

It's a member of the ivy family and grows in forests from Maine to the Midwest but is most abundant in the regions of the Appalachians and Ozarks.

How to Use: There are several ways you can take American Ginseng. You can eat its roots either raw or steamed. You can also make a tea or an infusion from the roots. Use about two grams of root for each cup of tea. If you're using powder, this would be the equivalent of one teaspoon. If you're using the root, you one or two medium-sized roots. Allow it to steep between 5 and 15 minutes, depending on the desired strength. Add any to taste.

Blackberry

This wonderfully delicious berry may be the answer to your inflammation. With a botanical name of *Rubus fruticosus*, Native Americans have employed the root-bark and leaves of the blackberry for a variety of physical conditions.

Blackberries grow in northern temperate areas and can be found in abundance on both the east and west coasts of North America.

How to Use: You can make a tincture out of the berries, or you can make blackberry tea or an infusion using the plants' leaves. Use two teaspoons of fresh leaves for each cup of water. Steep for about five minutes.

Buck Brush

The Cherokee called it Hummingbird Blossom and used it as an anti-inflammatory. Its botanical name is *Ceanothus,* with nearly 60 species native to North America, mostly in California and Oregon. The root of this plant holds its healing qualities.

How to Use: For the best results, make a tea from two teaspoons of the ground root for each cup of water, adjusting for your tastes. Steep it for about four minutes.

Skullcap

If you're looking for a natural way to reduce inflammation, you couldn't find a more effective herb than skullcap. A member of the mint family, its botanical name is *Scutellaria lateriflora* and grows abundantly throughout the northern United States. Sometimes it's referred to as Blue or Virginian Skullcap, Hoodwort, or Mad Dog.

How to Use: You can make a tincture using the leaves and flowers. You can also make a tea or infusion, using one tablespoon of fresh leaves or flowers for one cup of tea. Steep five to ten minutes, depending on the strength desired.

Yarrow

Native Americans employed yarrow as an anti-inflammatory as well as a remedy for other ailments. Its botanical name is *Achillea millefolium*, but you may hear people call it Nosebleed Plant, Old Man's Pepper, and even Devil's Nettle. It grows throughout North America.

How to Use: To prepare yarrow tea, add one teaspoon of the dried flower to a cup of water. Allow it to steep for 30 minutes. You can also make a tincture out of the leaves. To apply the herb topically, make a poultice from its leaves.

Insect Bites and Bee Stings

Honeysuckle

This plant has been cherished for centuries as a healing herb. All parts of the plant, from the stems to the juice and fruit, are used for a variety of remedies. Its botanical name is *Lonicera,* and North America is home to nearly two hundred species that grow in temperate regions.

How to Use: Make a salve of the leaves and flowers of this plant and apply it to the sting or bite.

Witch Hazel

You've probably used this for years to relieve the itching and pain of stings and bites. Instead of reaching for a bottle you bought in the store, trying to make your own. A shrub with the botanical name *Hamamelis virginiana*, it grows as far north as Canada and as far south as Texas and Florida.

How to Use: Prepare a tincture from the twigs and bark of the plant. Then apply it to the affected areas.

Insomnia

Chamomile

If you suffer from insomnia, then you're probably already

familiar with the relaxing qualities of chamomile. Instead of buying commercially prepared teas, why not try making your own from the fresh plant?

It has the botanical name *Matricaria chamomilla* and grows naturally in the northeastern region of the United States. You may find this hardy and invasive flower in other areas of the country as well.

How to Use: To prepare chamomile tea, use three to four tablespoons of the flowers for one cup of water. Steep this for five minutes. Drink it shortly before bedtime.

Hops

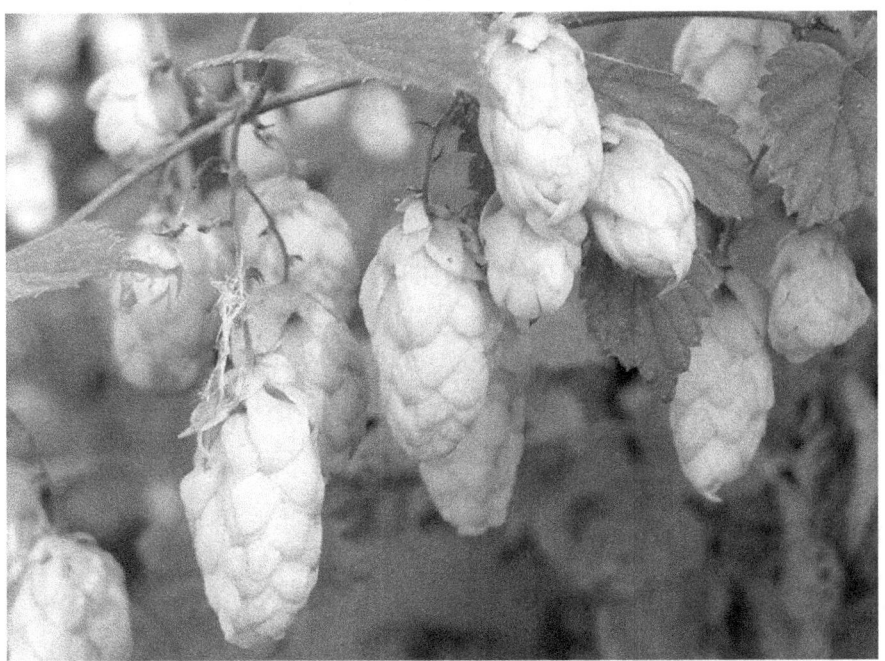

When you hear the word hops, does your first thought turn to beer? Beyond this traditional use, perhaps it's time to think of the relaxing powers this plant possesses in its own right. With the botanical name of *Humulus lupulus*, three varieties are native to North America and can be found in the southwestern and eastern regions as well as in the Midwest.

How to Use: Native Americans would fill a sachet with the herb inside a pillow to induce sleep. While you can do this or you can make tea from its flower cones. Use between two and five flowers for each cup of tea. Steep this between 20 and 30 minutes.

Passion Flower

Also known as Passion Vine, this herb was one the colonists quickly adopted from the Native Americans. Its scientific name is *Passiflora*; it's a valuable healing herb for several conditions, of which insomnia is one.

The passionflower grows from Ohio west to California and as far south as the Florida Keys.

How to Use: Prepare tea with either one tablespoon of dried leaves or two tablespoons of fresh for each cup of Passion Flower tea. Steep this for six to eight minutes.

Warning: Do not use this remedy if you are breastfeeding or pregnant.

Itching

Feverwort

This leafy plant with the scientific name *Triosteum perfoliatum* is a member of the honeysuckle family and was used by Native Americans to relieve itching. You'll probably know it as boneset, but it goes by other names as well, including Wild Coffee Fever-root and Tinker's Weed.

You can find it in the open, rocky woods and in thickets in the eastern United States from Massachusetts to Georgia. It's also found from Louisiana west to Oklahoma and from Nebraska to Minnesota.

How to Use: Apply a poultice made from the entire herb to the affected area or make a feverwort balm to place on the itching.

Stoneseed

Stoneseed can also relieve persistent itching. You may know it as Gromwell. With the botanical name of *Lithospermum officinale,* this herb grows in the western part of North America from California to western Colorado. Many Native Americans made a syrup from this herb to ease itching.

How to Use: Make a syrup from the decoction of the roots and stems of the stoneseed.

Kidney Health

Cattail

The cattail is probably not a plant you think of as having healing properties, but the Native Americans made use of all parts of it. And it's an aid to the health of your kidneys.

Its botanical name is *Typha,* and eleven species grow in the wetlands of the United States. The cattail also goes by the name Corndog Grass and Bullrush.

How to Use: Every part of this herb can be used to increase your kidney health. The roots can be cooked and eaten. You can grill, bake or boil them until they are tender.

The pollen, which is the spike at the top of the plant, is an amazing source of protein. Boil them for 10 to 12 minutes.

The corms are the small shoots and stubs that grow at the base of the cattail. Remove them from the rest of the plant and peel. You can eat these raw or cooked.

The spikes or stalks, which are the shoots of the plant, can be fried in butter or olive oil or can be eaten raw.

Goldenrod

The Native Americans used this herb with the botanical name *Solidago canadensis* or *Solidago virgaurea* for centuries. This plant is an abundant source of vitamin C.

How to Use: Prepare a goldenrod tea using two tablespoons of its fresh flowers for every cup of water. Allow it to steep about 15 minutes before serving. If you'd like, sweeten it with honey. You can also make a tincture with the flowers.

Laryngitis

American Licorice

There's a reason why licorice is an ingredient in cough drops; that's because it works. That's also the reason Native Americans used it as a remedy for laryngitis. This valuable herb, with the scientific name of *Glycyrrhiza lepidota*, grows naturally throughout the United States, with the exception of some southeastern areas.

How to Use: Prepare tea from the roots of the herb using one teaspoon of dried roots for each cup of water. Steep for two or three minutes. If you prefer, you can make a syrup.

Warning: Long-term use of licorice can cause fluid and electrolyte imbalances. If you have high blood pressure, heart disease, or are breastfeeding, you should consider using an alternative herbal remedy.

Mullein

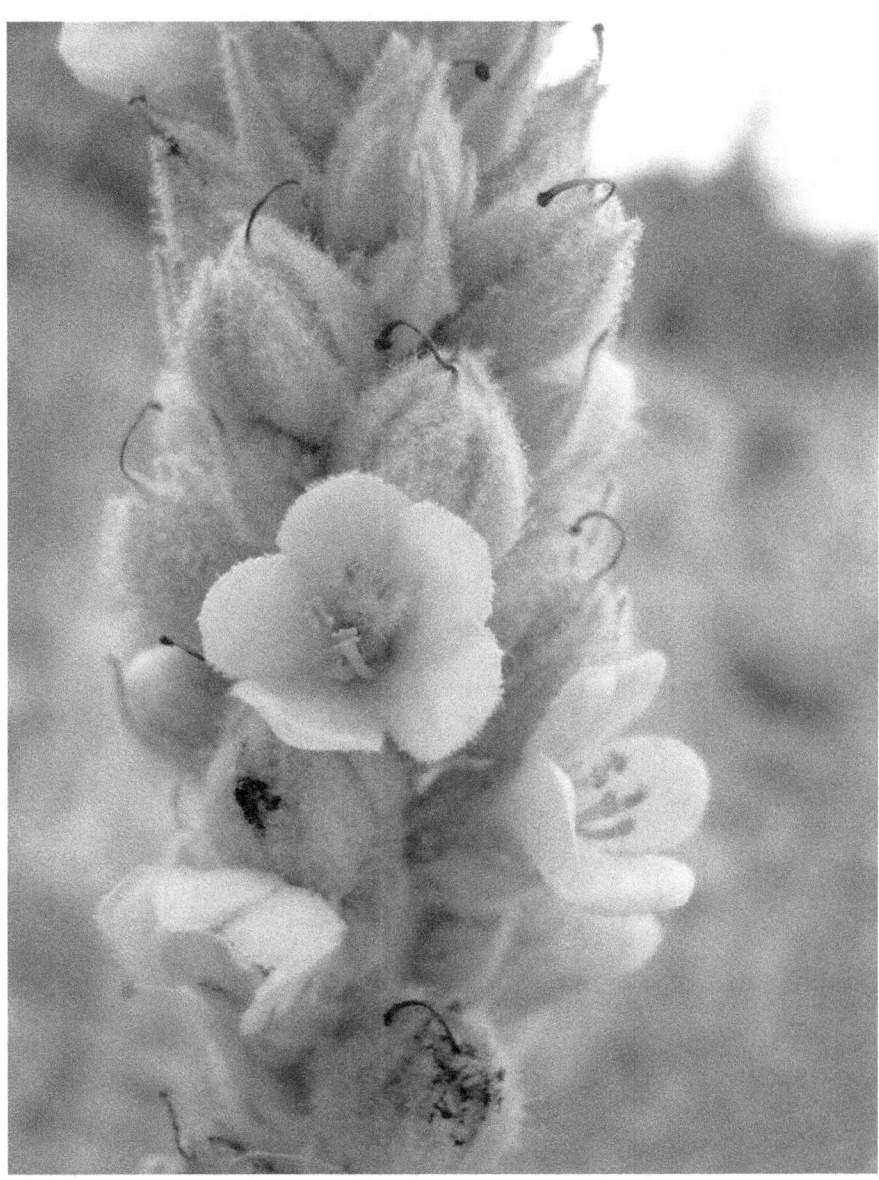

Mullein, with the scientific name of *Verbascum thapsus*, is also known as common mullein and is found nearly everywhere on the North American continent. Native Americans had multiple uses for this herb. The Creek tribe, for example, used it to treat coughs. It's also recommended as a remedy to treat laryngitis.

How to Use: Use a small handful of dried leaves for each cup of tea. Let this steep between five and 15 minutes, depending on strength. You can also make a syrup from it.

Slippery Elm

This tree, with the scientific name of *Ulmus rubra,* grows naturally in a variety of disparate areas in the United States. It can be found in the east and in southeast North Dakota as well as in northern Florida and eastern Texas.

The bark of this tree contains mucilage, which helps to calm inflamed or irritated tissue, making it the perfect remedy for laryngitis.

How to Use: Use approximately two tablespoons of the root powder for each cup of water. Allow it to steep for five minutes.

Liver Health

Dandelion

The lowly dandelion is an herbal remedy disguised as a weed. With the scientific name of *Taraxacum officinale*, this herb may be able to help keep your liver healthy. It possesses a host of phytonutrients and vitamins, including vitamins A, C, D, and B complex.

The Pillager Ojibwas and the Mohegan considered dandelion tea a health tonic and drank it daily.

How to Use: If you're making tea from the flowers, you'll use ten heads or flowers per cup of tea. Allow it to steep for up to 20 minutes. You can sweeten this with honey.

To make tea from the leaves, you'll use about six leaves, dried and finely chopped, for each cup of tea. Allow this to steep for about 10 minutes. Sweeten to taste.

If you use the root, either in fresh or dried form, you'll

only need two teaspoons of the taproot, chunked for each quart of tea. This needs to steep for about 40 minutes If you use dried root.

Goldenseal

Goldenseal is a popular supplement, and for a good reason. Its potency and medicinal properties were used by the Native Americans for centuries. With the botanical name *Hydrastis canadensis*, this herb is a member of the buttercup family. It goes by several names, including Orange Root, Yellow Root, or Ground Raspberry. Its native habitat is mostly in the eastern regions of the United States.

How to Use: To make a tea, use one teaspoon of the powdered root for each cup. Steep this for up to 20 minutes. If you make the tea from the herb's leaves, use one teaspoon and allow it to steep for three to six minutes. If the taste isn't to your suiting, the tea can be sweetened with honey or lemon.

Schisandra

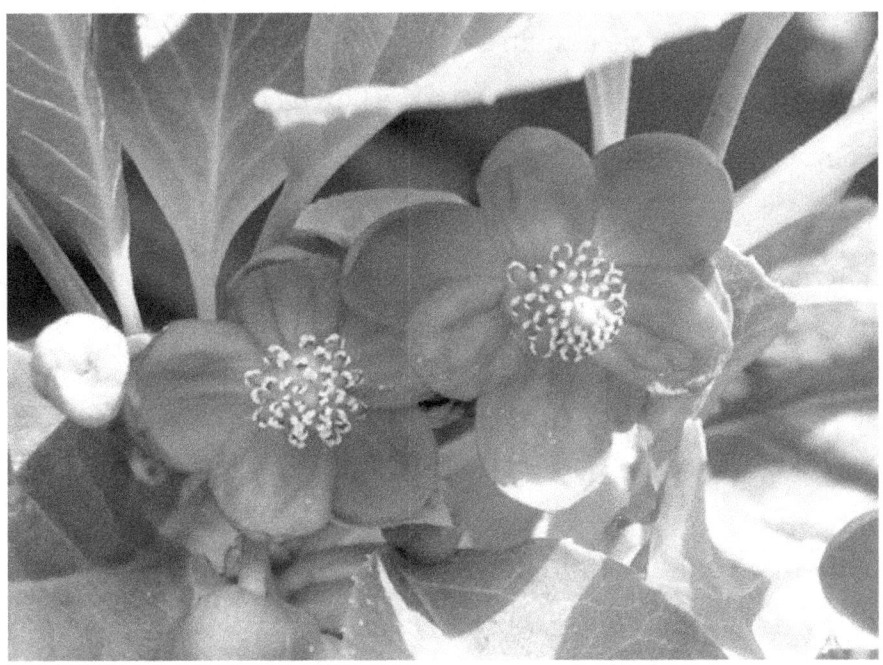

You may know this herb, which grows in the cooler climates of North America as Magnolia Vine. Its flowers have a delightful fragrance, and its berries are rich with phytonutrients, making them much loved by the Native Americans.

In addition to promoting live health, this herb can also help improve your mood and relieve fatigue.

How to Use: You can make a tea using one to two tablespoons of the dried berries for two cups of water. Using dried berries ensures as much phytonutrient content as possible is extracted. Allow it to steep between 15 and 20 minutes.

The dried berries can also be made into a tincture with a ratio of one part dried berries for six parts water.

Yellow Root

This plant makes its home in the eastern United States. Known botanically as *Rumex crispus*, it grows naturally from Maine to the northern part of Florida. It can be found as far west as Ohio and south to eastern Texas.

Native Americans used Yellow Dock as a blood purifier, and rightly so. Its phytonutrients stimulate liver activity.

How to Use: You can drink the tea made from its roots by using one tablespoon of the ground root for each cup of water. Allow it to steep for five minutes. Many people find the herb goes well when made in combination with another herb, particularly dandelion. Of course, you can always make a decoction out of this or a tincture as well.

Memory

American Ginseng

Like its cousin Asian ginseng, this herb historically has been used to aid in boosting memory. With the botanical name of *Panax Quinquefolius*, its home is in the forests of eastern North America.

How to Use: The best and most effective use of this herb is through use as a tea, tincture, or decoction. To make the tea, use about two ounces of the root for a cup of water. Allow it to steep for at least five and no more than 15 minutes.

Rosemary

Another herb known for its ability to increase your memory, Rosemary goes by the scientific name *Rosmarinus officinalis*. It's a member of the mint family and grows well in warm regions of the United States, such as California.

How to Use: To make rosemary tea, use about one teaspoon of the leaves for each cup. Allow it to steep between five and 15 minutes.

Menopausal Symptoms

Alfalfa

You may be surprised by this herb's use for menopausal symptoms. But alfalfa exhibits estrogen-like actions that are comparable to soy, the traditional herb of choice for these issues. With the botanical name of *Medicago sativa*, the alfalfa plant belongs to the pea family and is an abundant source of protein and calcium in addition to the B family of vitamins and vitamins E, C, and K.

How to Use: You can alfalfa sprouts to your salads or drink them as a tea. You can make alfalfa tea using either the dried leaves or the crushed seeds of the plant. If you the leaves, you'll need one teaspoon for each cup of water. Allow it to steep for ten to 15 minutes. If you choose to use the crushed-seeds method, you'll need one teaspoon of the seeds for every four cups of water. Allow this to boil for 30 minutes.

Black Cohosh

Native Americans depended on black cohosh as a remedy for a host of health issues, not the least of which were menopausal symptoms. Its scientific name is *Cimicifuga racemosa,* and it's native to the eastern regions of the United States. A member of the buttercup family, you may also hear it referred to as black bugbane, black snakeroot, or rattle weed.

How to Use: Make a tea from its roots using one teaspoon for each cup of water. Allow it to steep for about three minutes for a weak tea. If you want a stronger drink, you can steep it for up to 15 minutes. You may sweeten this to taste.

Sage

This is probably the mother of all healing herbs. Even if you're not familiar with herbal healing, you are more than likely aware of sage's potency. Burning sage is used by many to clear negative energy out of homes and other places. But one of its lesser-known abilities to help alleviate symptoms of menopause.

There are many species of sage in North America; one that was used by Native Americans was the white sage. Also referred to as bee sage or sacred sage, the botanical name of *Salvia apiana*. It grows naturally in the southwestern United States.

How to Use: To make tea, use two tablespoons of fresh common sage – or one tablespoon of dried leaves -- for each cup. Allow it to steep for three minutes.

St. John's Wort

The botanical name for St. John's Wort is *Hypericum perforatum*, but very often, people will call it Tipton's Weed, Chase Devil, and Klamath Weed. Native Americans used it for several ailments, but today it's been known to alleviate depression. It's also an excellent remedy for menopausal symptoms.

How to Use: Use two to three teaspoons of fresh flowers for every cup. Steep for about four minutes. You'll be delighted with its light lemony flavor.

Menstrual Pain and Cramps

Black Cohosh

In addition to its ability to alleviate menopausal symptoms, Black Cohosh can also help with cramps and other pain associated with your menstrual period. A member of the buttercup family, it carries the botanical name *Cimicifuga racemosa*. Black Cohosh is native to the eastern regions of North America.

How to Use: Use the roots of this plant to make a tea. You'll need one teaspoon of roots for each cup of water. For best results, it should steep for about 15 minutes. You can sweeten this if you'd like.

Partridgeberry

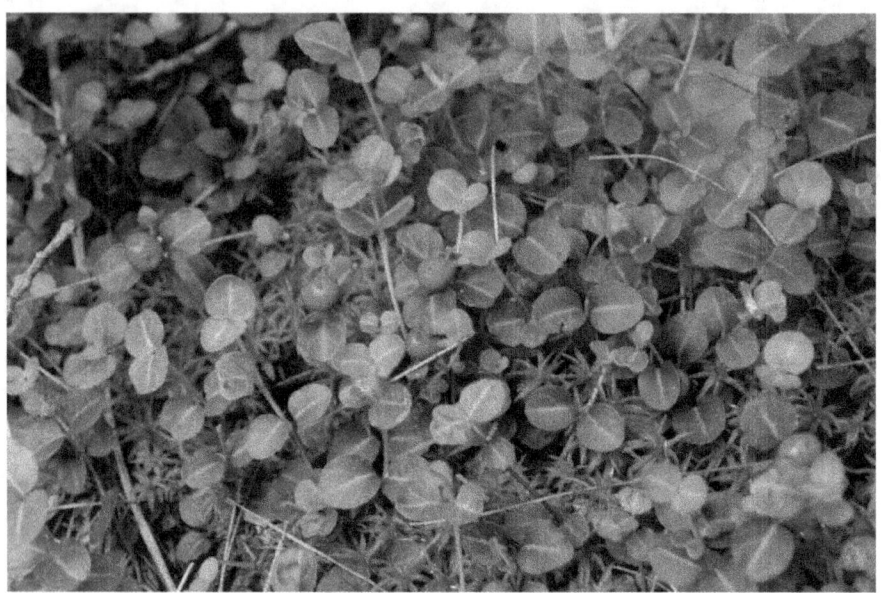

This herb, with the scientific name *Mitchella repens*, can be found in nearly every state and grows in wooded areas, along the banks of streams, and on sandy slopes. The Native Americans use this for a variety of reasons related to menstruation and pregnancy. The Cherokee drank tea made from the leaves in the final weeks of pregnancy to help ease the anticipated labor.

How to Use: You'll use the entire plant with the exception of the roots to make the tea. Use one teaspoon of the dried herbs for every cup of water. Allow it to steep for up to 15 minutes. You can drink this up to three times a day.

Sage

Just as this plant is an efficacious remedy for menopausal issues, it also helps to relieve the pain and cramping of menstruation. One of the native species of North America is white sage, *Salvia apiana*, which grows naturally in the southwestern regions of the United States.

How to Use: Use two tablespoons of the fresh sage leaves and one tablespoon of the dried leaves for each cup. Allow this to steep for about three minutes.

Menstrual Problems/Irregularities

Feverfew

Feverfew belongs to the sunflower family and has the botanical name *Tanacetum integrifolium*. This herb grows naturally throughout eastern North American and in Texas. Its native habitats are forest glades or open prairies. A species of the plant also grows in Arkansas.

In addition to using feverfew as a fever reducer, Native Americans employed it to help treat menstrual irregularities.

How to Use: You can make a tea with either dried or fresh petals. Use one cup of fresh petals for each cup of water. If you use dried petals, then you'll need two tablespoons per cup. Let it steep for approximately five minutes.

Partridgeberry

This herb grows in nearly every state in the union. You can find it in wooded areas, along the banks of streams, and on sandy slopes. It has the scientific name *Mitchella repens*.

Native Americans depended on this plant to treat a variety of menstrual problems, including irregularity.

How to Use: Make a tea using the entire plant except for its roots. You'll use one teaspoon of the dried herb for each cup of water. Let this steep for up to 15 minutes. You can drink three times a day if you like.

Sage

Just as Native Americans used sage to help relieve menopausal symptoms, they also employed it as a treatment for menstrual irregularities.

Many species of this plant can be found in North America, but one particularly stands out – white sage. With the botanical name *Salvia apiana*, this herb naturally grows in southwestern regions of the United States. Sometimes you'll hear it referred to as bee or sacred sage.

How to Use: Use two tablespoons of fresh sage for each cup of tea. If you're using dried leaves, use only one tablespoon. Let this steep for three minutes.

Morning Sickness

Raspberry

If you feel as if you're the first woman to experience morning sickness, take heart in knowing it plagued the Native Americans as well. One of the herbs they turned to for relief was raspberry – specifically the raspberry leaf.

With the scientific name *Rubus idaeus*, the raspberry is a member of the rose family and grows throughout the United States, especially on the edge of forests.

Even today, women turn to raspberry leaf tea to help alleviate the symptoms of morning sickness. Today we know that the leaves of the raspberry have the ability to tone the muscles of the pelvic floor and the uterus, making childbirth easier.

How to Use: For every cup of tea you make, use one to two teaspoons of the herb's dried leaves. Let this steep, covered, for about 10 minutes. You'll love the taste, but if you like, you can sweeten it.

Nettles

The leaves of the nettles plant, sometimes called stinging nettles, are rich in phytonutrients, which help to ease that nausea feeling first thing in the morning. This plant, with the botanical name of *Urtica dioica,* grows naturally everywhere in the continental United States.

How to Use: For every cup of tea, use one teaspoon of the

nettles leaves. This ratio remains the same for the dried leaves as well. Allow this to steep for about 10 minutes.

Ginger

The Native Americans knew the root of the wild ginger, scientifically called *Asarum canadense,* as a wonderful treatment for morning sickness. Ginger traditionally has been used to calm the stomach.

Ginger grows throughout North America. It grows along the Atlantic coast west to the Great Plains.

How to Use: Make a decoction of the thinly sliced root, using about one-half tablespoon for each cup. Allow this to steep between 15 to 30 minutes, depending on the strength you desire.

Chamomile

It's not surprising that Native Americans used chamomile, renowned for its calming abilities, to help alleviate the symptoms of morning sickness.

With the botanical name *Matricaria chamomilla*, this prized herbal remedy is native to the northeastern regions of North America.

How to Use: Use three to four tablespoons of the plant's flowers for each cup of water. Steep for three to five minutes.

Muscles

American Ginseng

You may be familiar with ginseng as a remedy for fatigue, but it's also a great herb to help with issues related to your muscles. With the botanical name, *Panax quinquefolius*, it's a member of the ivy family.

It grows naturally in forests as far east as Maine and throughout the Midwest, especially in the Appalachian region. It also grows in the Ozark region.

It's not only soothing to your sore muscles, but it may also help build muscle strength.

How to Use: Make a balm using the roots of this herb.

Evening Primrose

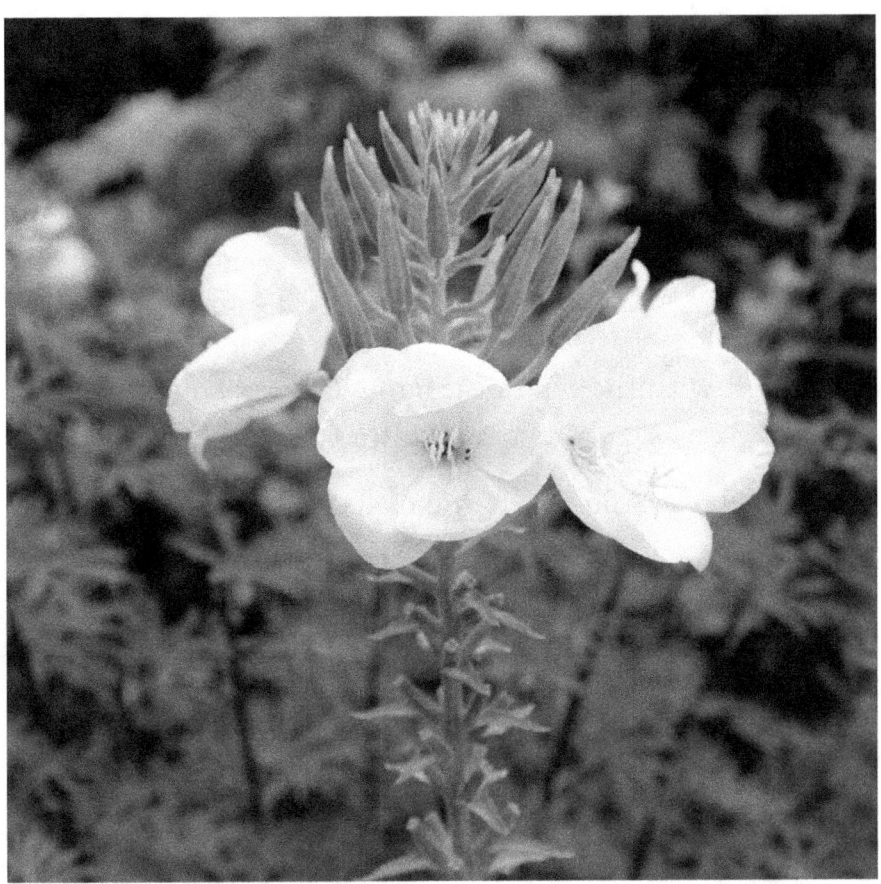

The Native Americans found the entire plant healing as they used different parts for various ailments, including muscle strain.

This herb's botanical name is *Oenothera biennis*, but you may have heard it called evening star, hogweed, or King's cure-all. The evening primrose grows naturally in the eastern and central areas of North American as well as Florida and Texas.

How to Use: Use the infused oil of the plant's flowers.

Greenbrier

This plant with the botanical name *Smilax bona-nox* is also known as Horsebrier and Bullbrier. This woody vine grows in the southeastern and eastern regions of the United States.

The Native Americans have used greenbrier as a remedy for at least a half-dozen conditions, including muscle pains and cramps.

How to Use: Use the entire plant, including the roots, as a poultice or a balm to place on the area affected.

Nausea

Chamomile

It's not surprising that this herb used to help you sleep better and alleviate morning sickness symptoms would also be a good remedy for nausea. This popular herb, which has the botanical name *Matricaria chamomilla*, grows naturally in the northeastern areas of North America.

How to Use: Make a tea using three to four tablespoons of the flowers for each cup of water. Steep for three to five minutes.

Feverwort

This is another Native American herb with many uses, one of which is to relieve nausea. Its botanical name is *Triosteum perfoliatum*, but you may have heard it called boneset. Feverwort belongs to the honeysuckle family and grows in the eastern regions of North America, especially in the thickets. It also grows from Louisiana as far west as Oklahoma and from Nebraska north to Minnesota.

How to Use: Use one tablespoon of the leaves and flowering tops for each cup of water. Steep this for 10 to 15 minutes.

Raspberry

Native Americans found the raspberry, which is botanically species *Rubus idaeus* and *rosaceae,* to be helpful in alleviating nausea. This herb grows throughout the United States.

How to Use: Use a ratio of two teaspoons of dried leaves for each cup of water. Allow this to steep for up to 10 minutes. Sweeten to taste.

Pain

Black Cohosh

Native Americans valued this herb as a pain reliever. With the botanical name *Cimicifuga racemosa*, this plant grows abundantly throughout the eastern United States. Some people call it rattle weed, fairy candle, or black snakeroot.

How to Use: Make a poultice using its roots.

Evening Primrose

This is one of Native Americans' all-purpose herb and a valuable one for pain. Botanists refer to it as *Oenothera biennis*, but laymen regularly call it evening star, hogweed, and King's cure-all. You'll find it in abundance throughout the eastern and central areas of North America. The evening primrose also grows in Florida and Texas.

How to Use: The most effective use is the application of infused oils using the flowers.

Skullcap

The Native Americans used this herb to help reduce inflammation, which is the cause of all pain. This member of the mint family has the botanical name *Scutellaria lateriflora* and grows throughout the northern United States. Don't be surprised to hear some individuals call it Blue or Virginian Skullcap, Hoodwort, or Mad Dog.

How to Use: You can use this as an infused oil of the leaves and flowers to apply to the affected area.

PMS

Black Cohosh

Once again, Black Cohosh tops the list of most effective herbal remedies. This time for the symptoms of PMS. You may encounter it as black snakeroot, fairy candle, or rattle weed, but all of these refer to the same plant, botanically called *Cimicifuga racemosa*.

How to Use: For one cup of tea, use one teaspoon for the dried root. Let it steep for up to three to 15 minutes, depending on the strength you need. Sweeten to taste.

Chamomile

This calming tea is one of the best choices if you suffer from PMS.

Chamomile, which resembles the daisy, grows throughout the United States and is especially prevalent in the northeast. Its scientific name is *Matricaria chamomilla*.

How to Use: For each cup of water, use three to four tablespoons of fresh flowers. Steep for three to six minutes.

Pneumonia

Dogwood

This historically has been the Native American go-to herbal treatment for pneumonia. With the scientific name *Cornus florida*, it's also known as American Dogwood or Boxwood. The tree grows from Maine to Florida on the east coast, in Texas and several midwestern states, including Minnesota and Kansas.

How to Use: Use only the dried bark for the infusion. Fresh bark will only make your stomach and bowels feel worse. Steep one tablespoon in a pint of water for about 30 minutes.

Pleurisy Root

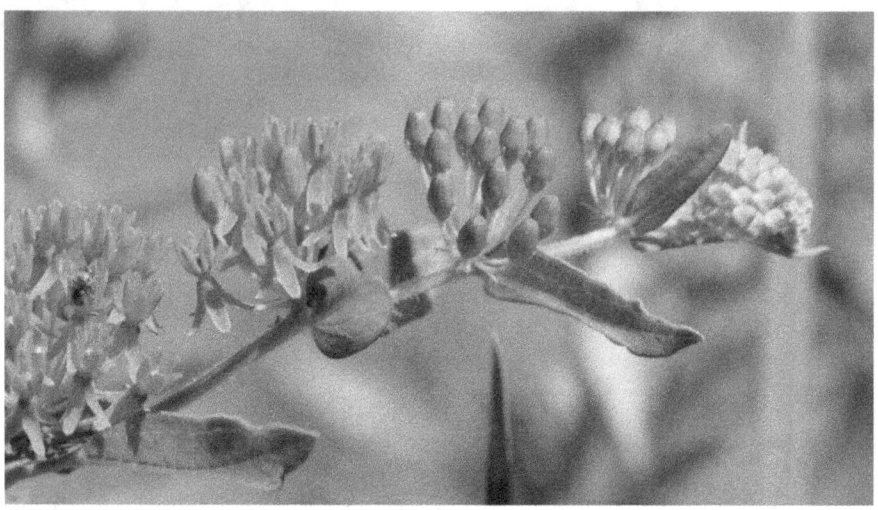

This aptly named herb has been used for centuries by Native Americans for a variety of respiratory issues, including pneumonia. It has the scientific name *Asclepias tuberosa,* and it a member of the milkweed family. Found in eastern North American, pleurisy root also goes by the name of Butterfly Weed, Flux Root, and Orange Milkweed.

The Natchez people drank a tea made from the root of this herb as a remedy for pneumonia.

How to Use: For each pint of water, use one teaspoon of

the dried root, chopped. Allow this to steep for up to 15 minutes. A tincture of the fresh root also can be used.

Warning: Pleurisy root should not be used by pregnant women.

Rabbit Tobacco

This plant may have an amusing name, but it's a seriously good remedy to help you get through the symptoms of pneumonia. It grows naturally throughout the eastern region of North America in open, dry sandy ground.

Botanists refer to it as *Gnaphalium obtusifolium*, but you may hear it called sweet everlasting or old field balsam. You can recognize it nearly instantly due to its sweet maple syrup-like aroma.

How to Use: Make an infusion using one teaspoon of the leaves and flowers for each cup of water. Let this steep for five minutes.

Wild Black Cherry

Native Americans called this plant Chokecherry, and botanists call it *Prunus serotina*. They used it for a variety of respiratory ailments, including pneumonia. You can find it throughout the United States.

How to Use: Make a tincture using the bark and take 10 drops a day.

Poison Ivy, Oak, or Sumac

Sumac

You may find it counterintuitive to use sumac to help heal poison sumac, but the Native Americans successfully used this remedy. Sumac grows throughout North America. Its botanical name is *Rhus glabra*, but you'll also hear it referred to as Dwarf, Mountain, or Scarlet Sumac. Native Americans used this regularly for poison ivy and other skin eruptions.

How to Use: Place a poultice of the leaves and berries on the affected area.

Witch Hazel

In addition to being a great remedy for burns, it can also help relieve poison ivy. Witch Hazel is a shrub that is known as *Hamamelis virginiana* to botanists. It grows from northern Canada to Texas and Florida.

How to Use: Either a poultice from the twigs and bark of the plant, or you can make a tincture and apply it to the affected area.

Prostate Conditions

Prickly Pear Cactus

Though this plant is a cactus, it grows throughout the United States. With the scientific name, *Opuntia engelmannii*, the prickly pear cactus and was part of the Native American diet in addition to an herbal remedy.

How to Use: Use one-and-half teaspoons of the berries for each cup of tea. Steep this for about four minutes.

Saw Palmetto

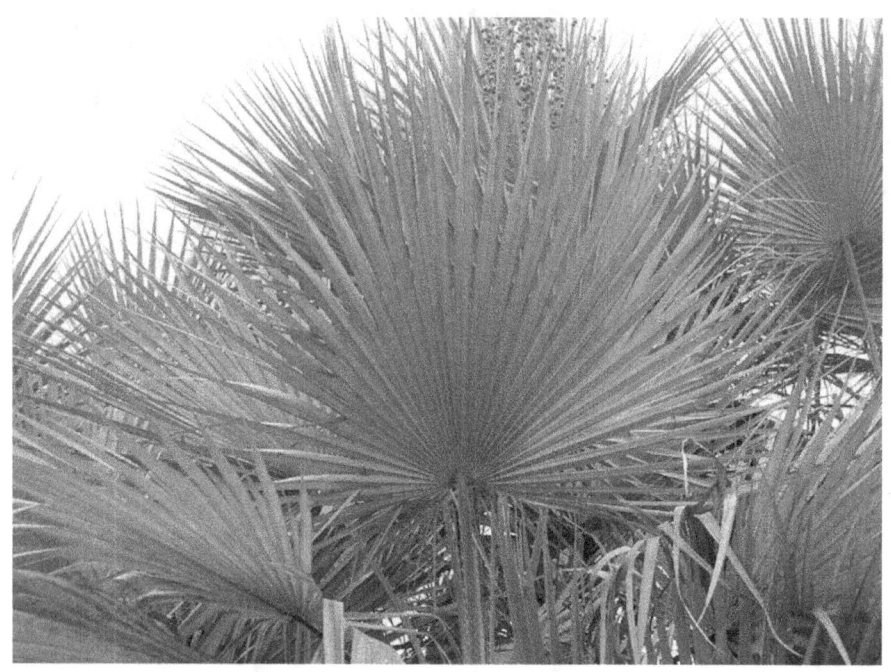

Native Americans used this small palm tree for a variety of herbal remedies as well as part of their daily diet. With a botanical name of *Serenoa serrulata*, this tree grows throughout the southeastern United States. Its berries are prized for their ability to help alleviate enlarged prostate.

How to Use: Use a one-quarter cup of fresh berries or two teaspoons of dried berries for two cups of tea. Steep this for three to six minutes. You may sweeten to taste.

Horsetail

It's more widely known as a pain-reliever, but horsetail also remedies prostate issues. You may hear it called Shavegrass, scouring rush, or even bottle brush, but they all refer to the plant *Equisetum arvense*. Horsetail grows abundantly along the banks of streams and in the meadows throughout the United States.

How to Use: Use one handful of the entire herb with the exception of the roots for every two cups of water. Allow this to steep for 15 minutes.

Respiratory Problems

Slippery Elm

The Native Americans used slippery elm inner bark to treat a variety of respiratory issues.

This tree grows in various regions of the country. You can find it in the eastern United States as well as in the southeast region of North Dakota. It also is native to northern Florida as well as eastern Texas.

How to Use: For each cup of water, use two tablespoons of bark powder. Allow this to steep for about five minutes.

Wild Onion

Similar to its cousin garlic, the wild onion possesses a myriad of healing compounds, some of which can aid in respiratory issues. It's a member of the Allium family with nearly 600 species scattered throughout the United States – all of them with the same healing powers.

How to Use: To make wild onion tea, use half of a large onion for each cup. Steep for three to five minutes. You may need to sweeten it with honey.

Restless Legs Syndrome or Restless Sleep

Chamomile

This is the go-to Native American herb for any type of sleep problems, even those related to restless leg syndrome.

Chamomile, known to botanists as *Matricaria chamomilla*, is native to northeastern North America. It grows so abundantly; in fact, it's known as an invasive flower.

How to Use: Take three to four tablespoons of the flowers for each cup of tea. Steep for three to six minutes.

Hops

This plant, known as an ingredient in beer, is also a remedy for restless leg syndrome. The botanical name for this plant is *Humulus lupulus,* and three varieties of it grow in the United States. You can find this herb in the southwestern, eastern, and Midwest regions of the United States.

How to Use: Make a tea from two to five flower cones for each cup of tea. Allow it to steep for about five minutes.

Skullcap

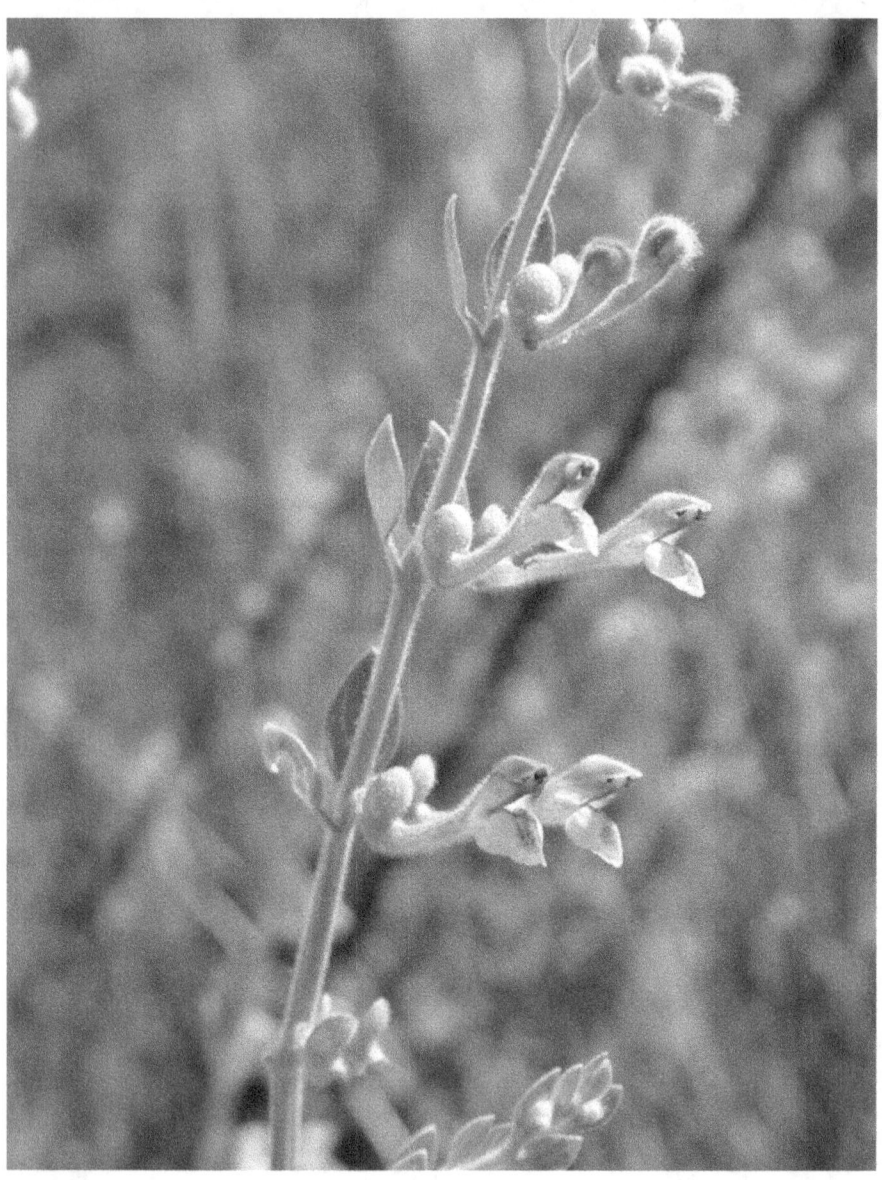

Native Americans used the member of this mint family

for a variety of ailments, and today we find it helps to relieve restlessness with the botanical name *Scutellaria lateriflora*. It grows throughout the northern region of the United States and depending on who you talk with, it's called Blue or Virginian Skullcap, Hoodwort, or Mad Dog.

How to Use: To make tea from skullcap's fresh flowers or leaves, use one tablespoon for each cup of water.

How to Use: You can make a tincture using the leaves and flowers. You can also make a tea or infusion, using one tablespoon of fresh leaves or flowers for one cup of tea. Steep for five to ten minutes.

Rheumatoid Arthritis

Broom Snakeweed

You may hear this plant referred to as simply snakeweed, but it's still the same plant botanists call *Gutierrezia sarothrae*. The Navajo employed this herb regularly for pain.

It grows in the western states in arid climates as well as

the mountains.

How to Use: Use as poultice or salve using the entire plant except for its roots. You can also make a tea with tea teaspoons of the herb to one cup of water. Steep five to 10 minutes.

Indian Hemp

The Native Americans used this variety of marijuana for various kinds of pain. Its botanical name is *Apocynum cannabinum*, but you may also hear people call it dogbane, Amy root, or Rheumatism root.

It grows naturally throughout North America in gravelly or sandy soil and near streams.

How to Use: You'll need one teaspoon of dry hemp leaves for each cup of water. Allow it to steep for three to five minutes. Hemp isn't water-soluble, so it's recommended you add some milk.

Sedative/Soothing agent

Chamomile

The Native Americans knew chamomile could relax your system and soothe your nerves. You probably know it best as a sleeping aid.

With the botanical name *Matricaria chamomilla*, this herb grows abundantly in the northeast United States.

How to Use: To make one cup of chamomile flower tea, use three to four tablespoons of the fresh flowers. Steep for three to six minutes.

Rabbit Tobacco

This plant, also called sweet everlasting by some herbalists for its sweet maple-syrup like aroma, may have a calming effect on you.

Its botanical name is *Gnaphalium obtusifolium*, but it also goes by field balsam. You can find it growing in dry, sandy ground throughout the eastern United States.

How to Use: Make a tea or infusion with one teaspoon of the leaves and flowers for each cup of water. Allow this to steep for about five minutes.

Skullcap

This herb is best known for its pain-relieving properties, but it possesses calming qualities as well.

The botanists call this member of the mint family *Scutellaria lateriflora,* and it grows throughout the northern United States. You may hear it referred to as Blue or Virginian Skullcap or even Mad Dog.

How to Use: To make one cup of tea, use a teaspoon of the leaves and flowers. Let it steep for up to 15 minutes.

Sinus Problems

American Ginseng

If you like me, you associate this herb with a remedy for fatigue, but Native Americans used it as other remedies as well, including sinus issues.

The botanical name is *Panax quinquefolius* and grows in the forests of eastern North America.

How to Use: For each cup of the infusion you make, use about four tablespoons of the root. Allow it to steep for 15 minutes.

Garlic

The herb garlic, or Allium sativum, is one we're all familiar with. But you may not have realized it was an excellent sinus remedy. The Native Americans relied on garlic for a variety of issues, including colds and flu.

How to Use: You can make garlic juice by crushing five fresh cloves and straining the juice.

Or you can create an infused steam of garlic. Add five crushed cloves of fresh garlic to a pot of boiling water. Drape a towel over your head and bend over the pot. Deeply inhale the steam. Do this for several minutes or until you can feel the remedy working.

Goldenseal

This member of the buttercup family may be the alternative to over-the-counter sinus medications you've been searching for.

It has the botanical name *Hydrastis canadensis* but also goes by Orange or Yellow Root and Ground Raspberry. Goldenseal flourishes in the eastern regions of North America.

How to Use: To make a tea from the ground leaves, use one teaspoon to two cups of water. Use the same amount of the root for an infusion. Allow it to steep for three to six minutes.

Warning: Goldenseal should not be taken by pregnant women.

Sage

Native Americans held this herb in high esteem for its purifying effects, and that extends to the sinuses.

Several species grow in the southwestern United States. The most common of these has the botanical name *Salvia apiana*, or white sage. It's also called bee or sacred sage.

How to Use: Two tablespoons of fresh sage or one tablespoon of the dried herb is used for each cup of tea. Allow it to steep for three to five minutes.

Wounds

Garlic

Twentieth-century medicinal research has confirmed what the Native Americans knew all along – that garlic facilitates the healing of wounds. Native American herbal healers couldn't tell you that this bulb contained antibiotic and antimicrobial qualities, but nevertheless, they knew it worked.

Garlic can quickly quell the pain, help to stop bleeding as well as hasten healing. But this aromatic herb does double duty because it also helps protect your wound from infection.

How to Use: Make a poultice of crushed garlic cloves.

Aloe Vera

We mentioned this herb before when we talked about burns. Native Americans relied on this herb for all types of skin issues. Its botanical name is *Aloe barbadensis miller* and grows in the warmer climates of the United States.

How to Use: Carefully slit open one of the leaves and apply the gel inside to the area affected. Once it dries, wash the area with warm water and pat it dry.

Onion

It should come as no surprise that the onion, garlic's cousin, is also an effective remedy for wounds. This plant has many phytonutrients that contribute to its effectiveness.

How to Use: Mix crushed onion with honey and use it as a paste to be applied directly to the wound.

Chapter 6: How to Become Your Own Herbal Healer

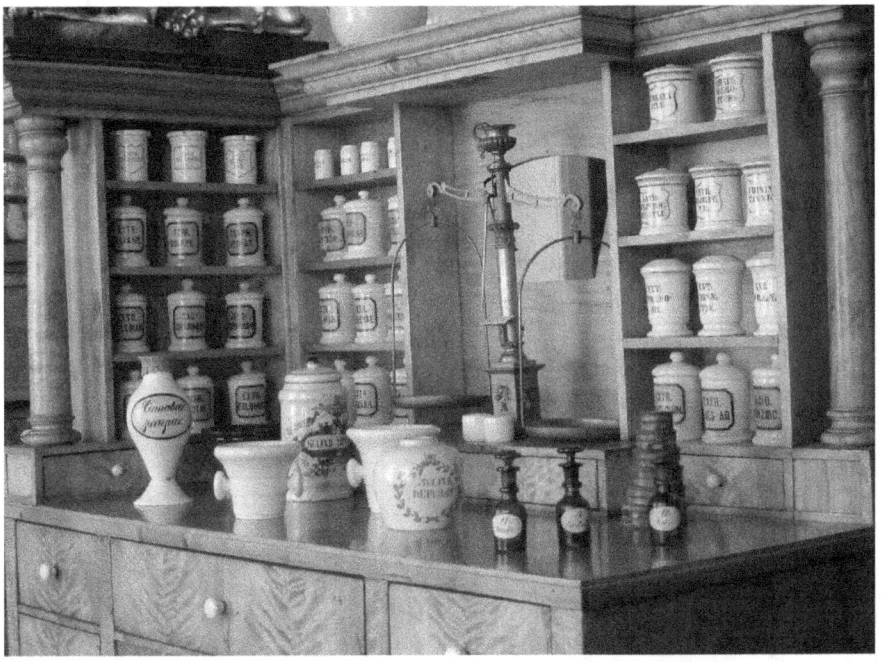

If you're even half as excited as I was when I realized the power of healing herbs, then you probably can't start practicing personal herbalism soon enough. And if you're anything like I was when I began, you're probably wondering how to get started. I had the advantage of watching Grace and taking inventory of everything she did and used.

You might not have the same luxury. But don't despair.
Even if you don't have a mentor, this portion of the book
will walk you through the essentials of becoming your
own herbalist. And as with any new endeavor, there are
several paths.

The key to any good journey, however, is not to expect to
get to your destination overnight. As you learn more
about the topic, you'll keep asking yourself, "Am I there
yet?" The answer to that is that you never really arrive.
Herbalism is a lifelong education in itself. There's always
more to learn. Always another path to take in the journey.
As with life itself, the pleasure and satisfaction lie in the
journey and not the destination.

If the idea of using healing herbs is new to you, then you
should take baby steps. I know this might not seem like
an exciting start, but by doing so, you'll be getting a solid
foundation from which to build.

Then you may be surprised to know you've already
started. Yep. You took your first step when you started

reading this book. And don't let this be the only volume you read on herbs. There are plenty out there. Familiarize yourself with as many of them as you can afford. Build yourself a reference library of herb books.

Growing Herbs

While you're building your library, you can take the next baby step of growing your own herbs. This can be as elaborate as a large plot of land in your backyard with a crazy variety of plants for many ailments. Or it could be a small window herb garden in your home. The choice is yours depending on your level of comfortableness with the idea.

Perhaps, you are already growing herbs for culinary purposes. I know Grace always had parsley available not only for healing but to throw into her delicious soups as well. Every time I visited her, I always left with a handful of parsley or basil. If you are already growing these, then you're a budding herbalist already.

What you decide to grow will depend on a few factors. If you're considering an outside garden, then you need to find out what will thrive in your climate. If you can't get the answers you need from an online search, then call your local county extension service. You can find them by searching online or by calling a local university.

Once you know what herbs to grow, then you need to increase your chances of success by seeking out advice on the soil, sunlight, and other growth requirements.

Tools You'll Need

Thankfully, the art of herbal healing is simple, which means the tools of your trade are simple as well. The best part of this is, you probably have most of them already in your home. The ones you don't already own can be bought fairly inexpensively.

Scissors and Baskets

I list these two as one because you'll find them to be practically inseparable when you harvest your herbs or when you forage. The scissors are for clipping the plants, and the baskets are for carrying your finds.

The scissors should be as high as quality as you can afford. The stems of some plants grow quite thick. You'll want to get as clean a cut as possible, and a small, inferior pair won't do the job.

And the baskets? Use your imagination with this tool. You will want it to have handles, and the size will depend on your trip. And don't think they need to be bought brand new. On your future trips to thrift stores, keep an eye on baskets. Every time I go into a thrift store, I make a beeline to the baskets – and then the canning jars. I have a collection of baskets that I choose. It makes a fun hobby even more delightful.

Mesh Sieve

This will become your most useful tool of all. Mine is. I have three of them, all different sizes. You can start with one. The finer the holes, the better. Just as with the baskets, it's hard to conceive of having too many sieves.

Potato Ricer

It's true, if odd, an odd necessity for an herbal student.

But a potato ricer is indispensable. I use this instead of the more expensive tincture press. The press and my ricer both apply pressure to the tincture to remove all of the liquid from the herbs.

Mortar and Pestle

Here is a utensil that you may initially associate with a pharmacist, but it's useful for an herbalist as well. If you're an avid cook, you may already have one of these in your kitchen. If not, it's not only essential to your herbal journey, it's also a beautiful addition to your décor. The mortar and pestle is the best method I've found for getting a coarse ground to herbs.

Spice Grinder

Any type of grinder you're comfortable with works. The best way to use herbs, of course, is fresh, and it's also best to wait to grind them on demand. If you're growing your own, this is one big advantage. You can be sure they'll freshly ground. If you don't already own one, there are plenty of types to choose from. And just like the baskets and the sieves, you may want to start your search at a thrift store.

Canning Jars

My canning jars are very useful. I saw how Grace used them for storing nearly everything from her dried herbs to her infused oils. She kept tea blends in them. Heck, she even made herbal sun tea in them. You'll need a good half-dozen to start.

Kitchen Scale

As you progress with your herbal education, you'll find some of the ingredients in recipes and formulas will be given in weights. This is especially true as you incorporate more herbs into your daily cooking. It's also a great device to have to give a more precise measurement of your teas and the potency of your tinctures.

Stainless Steel Canning Funnel

You'll need a funnel for those times you transfer your herbal recipes into mason jars. That will happen often. Guaranteed. If you've ever used a canning funnel, then you know they have a wider mouth than regular ones.

The mouth of the one I use is about five-and-a-half inches wide. It works wonderfully when I transfer either liquid concoctions or more solid recipes.

Tea Press

Like my potato ricer, this is one of my favorite herbal instruments. It makes brewing large amounts of tea so much easier. It's also great to use when you make infusions. If all you have at home is a coffee press, then use that. It serves the same purpose. But just a word of caution is in order. It's best to have one that's dedicated to your herbal avocation. That way, your teas won't have any lingering coffee taste.

Tea Strainer

A tea strainer is a perfect appliance for when you only require one cup of tea.

Electric Teapot

A teapot is a teapot, you may think. Before I immersed myself in herbs, I thought the same thing. But, believe me, this is very useful to have on hand, especially if you're making several batches of tea at a time. It heats the tea incredibly fast, and that's a quality you'll be grateful for.

Not to overwhelm you, but there are a few more utensils you'll need along your path to working with herbs. These, though, are guaranteed to be in your kitchen in some form right now. The items you have in your kitchen will serve you well for the moment. There may come a time, though, when you'll want to have dedicated tools for herbalism.

Knife

Just as with your scissors, you'll want to have sharp knives.

Cutting Board

A good cutting board isn't just a cook's best friend; it's also an herbalist's. You find that if you maintain a good quality cutting board, your preparations for your remedies will go much smoother.

Double Boiler

I probably don't need to tell you how great double boilers are. Even before I started using them for my herbal recipes and formulas, I used them when I made chocolate. A double boiler takes the worry out of burning the fragile herbs.

Don't have one right away? Take a large saucepan, fill it nearly half-way with water and sit a smaller one with the herbs on top of that. Viola! You're the owner of a double boiler.

Measuring Spoons

The ones you have for your baking are perfect for your herbal needs. Stainless steel spoons are the most desirable, but if all you have on hand as you start your herbal journey, then they'll work fine.

Glass Measuring Cups

Remember that thrift store visit for baskets? Put glass measuring cups on that list. You can never have too many. As you progress on your path in herbalism, you'll discover you'll need them in just about every size for your recipes. Not only that, when you strain your tinctures or oils, it will be much easier and less messy with the wonderful "spout" of the cup.

Large Mixing Bowls

I have only one word to describe their use: indispensable.

When you don't have your basket handy, these large bowls make a great substitute receptacle as you snip off the herbs. This is also the place you'll be combining your mixed herbal teas.

Surrounded by your budding herb garden and your gaggle of utensils, you've taken the first necessary steps to become your own herbalist. But there's more to learn. In the next chapter, we'll talk about the alternative option to growing herbs – foraging responsibly for them in the wild.

Chapter 7: How to Wildcraft

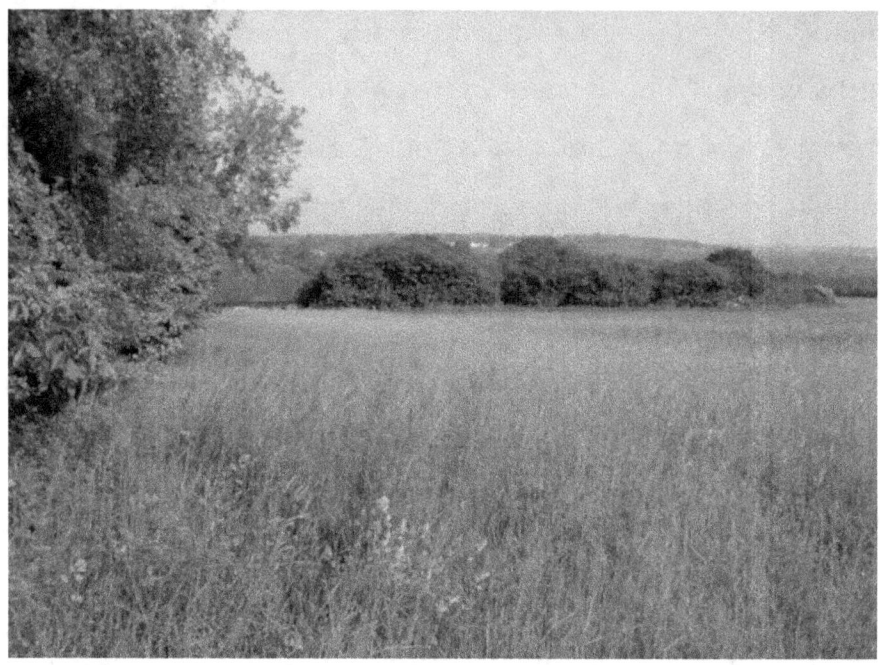

Foraging or an herb garden? Are you torn by choice? Don't be. Because you can do both quite easily. An herb garden provides you with the ease of accessibility to your most used herbs, that daily one for destressing, healing injuries, or alleviating your daily aches and pains.

Because you grow your own herbs doesn't mean you can't go on an occasional foraging adventure. Foraging, which is nothing more than discovering and harvesting plants in the wild, doesn't have to be intimidating. It can be as simple as going into a meadow and searching for clover or daisies.

When you forage for your herbs, you're wildcrafting. It's the process of gathering herbs in their natural environment. The herbs or dried herbs you buy from stores, even health food stores, were not grown in their natural environment unless it explicitly indicates this on the packaging.

And many herbalists believe responsible wildcrafting has two advantages. The first is the herbs more powerful when grown in their natural environment. Instead of being bred for sale, these herbs are receiving nutrients from the soil naturally. Getting nutrients through natural means is also better for your health and wellbeing.

The other advantage, though, involves your relationship with Mother Nature. It's something Grace would tell me. Wildcrafting for the herbs you need at the moment, and no more renews humanity's relationship with nature. As you forage, you'll look upon these plants as friends and allies in your healing, not merely as a product to be used.

Because Grace saw herbs this way, she always asked permission of the plant before harvesting it. This concept sounds wild and woo-woo to many westerners, but even today, the best wildcrafters practice this courtesy.

It may take you some time before you feel the connection with the plant world that Grace did, but it's there. It took me some months of wildcrafting with my friend before I felt that connection. At first, it seemed slight and far away, but as I spent more time with the plants, the relationships grew.

Rituals for Wildcrafting

Grace's sacred ritual for wildcrafting was simple yet powerful. She would sit with the flower she chose and watched it. She immersed herself in its environment through a short meditation. During that quiet period, she would ask permission from the plant. I asked her how she knew if the plant allowed her to harvest it. She answered me in the fashion of someone attuned to nature. "I can feel it," she would tell me.

Then she gently took what she needed — no more. Before she moved on, though, she paused for a few moments to thank the plant for its generosity. She would whisper a thank you or, at times, just smile down at it. She told me the plants understood her purpose.

And, yes, even before you ask, there were times the plant didn't agree to the arrangement. In those times, Grace sat in meditation and was denied the harvest; she never took it personally, and most importantly, she never got angry. And she never harvested it. She found another individual plant.

When you practice wildcrafting in this fashion, you can be assured of the herb's healing potency, not only because of its nutrient value but also because of the value of the relationship with it.

Now that you know the essentials of what wildcrafting is, here are some useful ideas to keep in mind before, during, and after your trip.

Be Able to Identify Herbs

The first rule of wildcrafting is knowing what you're looking at. In other words, you need to be proficient at identifying plants. And not just herbs. You should have a rudimentary knowledge of weeds, bushes, and trees. You should learn how to spot a plant by its leaves by the appearance of its fruit or berries.

In other words, study as much as you can before you leave your home. There are plenty of online resources and a myriad of field books to help you learn everything you need for a successful and safe wildcrafting experience.

This is the first rule because you don't want to harvest a dangerous doppelganger plant unaware. At best, using it could lead to mild discomfort. At worst, it could kill you.

Bring the Proper Tools

Prepare for your excursion, even if you only plan to spend a short time. You'll want to take either a pair of scissors with you or a pocket knife. I know some herbalists take a pair of small pruning shears if they are searching for larger plants. The cutting tools you take will depend on your potential harvest. But if you find an herb you weren't searching for but think will help you, you may want to carry a variety of tools.

Whatever you do, don't tear or rip the plant. You'll want the clean cut of a utensil. For one thing, a clean cut will help spur new growth. The purpose of wildcrafting is to preserve the environment. Ripping parts off plants defeats that purpose.

If you're foraging for roots, then don't forget to pack a small gardener's trowel. If you're going to be gone long, instead of taking a basket, you may want to take a box of sandwich-size plastic bags for temporary storage.

And lastly, always pack yourself a bottle of water and perhaps some snacks and don't forget a small first-aid kit.

Harvest with Permission

While you need the permission of the plant, you also need the consent of the owner of the private land. Before you go, research the area you plan on harvesting from. If it's private, check with the owner before embarking. If it's federal land, be sure harvesting is allowed.

Steer Clear of Highly Trafficked Areas

Once you do have consent, then you need to search for herbs that are as natural as possible, with as little human or animal influence as possible. The best herbs are at least 50 feet from any roadways. This way, you're assured that no stray animal or even a stray human has done their part in fertilizing them. The plant can easily retain any residue of the object, which in turn can be transferred to your preparation.

Harvest With the Welfare of the Plants in Mind

When you harvest parts from any group of plants, you should never take more than 20 percent of them. That's what responsible wildcrafting is all about. If you take more than that percentage, the odds increase that the plants can be damaged or be placed in shock, or even die. If there are five plants, only take what would be 20 percent of a plant. This may mean taking a leaf from several herbs instead of depleting an entire plant.

The concept behind this is harvesting to the needs of the plants. While foraging, consider what the plant or the community of plants needs to live. Don't take so much as to destroy the plant or injure the community.

You will also want to look around at where they're growing. If you find an invasive weed that you know will damage the plants, remove it for them. If there are broken branches around that may impede their growth, remove them as well. The plants will appreciate it.

Wildcraft only During the Plants' Growing Season

The concept behind this activity is respecting the plants. That includes their environment, of course, but it also means to respect their life cycles. Don't harvest when a plant can't continue to grow; that action isn't in line with the ideals and purpose of wildcrafting.

To follow this rule of thumb, you should be knowledgeable when it's best to harvest certain parts. When you honor their life cycles, you'll reap the benefits in addition to the plant. During their cycles, various portions of the plant will hold the most nutrients and are available at their peak at different times of the year.

For example, the leaves of most plants are the most tender in the spring, before the flowers bloom, and are, for the most part, haven't been exposed to insects. Once the flowers bloom; however, the leaves get tough, sometimes tasteless or even bitter. As a wildcrafting rule of thumb, it's always best to harvest leaves at their brightest in color.

When you're wildcrafting for flowers, there is, most naturally, a more obvious limited window of opportunity. Harvest the flowers that have most recently opened. If they've wilted, they're lacking in the phytonutrients you need for effectiveness.

If you're searching for buds, try timing your visit into the woods or meadows right before they open.

Wildcrafting roots are a different story. In this case, you should harvest them as late as possible prior to the first frost. This is a perfect time because it matches the life cycle of the plant. Its energy is receding into the ground as it prepares for winter. If you dig the roots after a frost, you may find them damaged and spongey. If you do wildcraft roots, there is a different rule of thumb for the amount to take. Instead, take no more than 10 percent of the community and less if you can.

If your formulas and recipes call for seeds, you'll receive the most benefit from them when you harvest while they're ripe. The seeds should be left on the plant so the sun can ripen them as long as possible, but before the wind flings them to other places. It is a delicate balancing act, but if you can time it correctly, it's worth the trouble.

You can tell when the seeds are ready by the condition of the stem. If the stem is dry, it's ready for wildcrafting. Collect them carefully. The method Grace taught me is the easiest one I've found. Put a paper bag around the plant and cut the stem; always leave the majority of the seeds for replenishment next year.

If you want to gather bark, you have your choice of times, either in the spring or in the fall. The best way to harvest bark is to take it from the recently fallen branches. Never take it from the trunk of the tree and never harvest more than 10 percent of its circumference.

Wildcraft in the Morning

The ideal time to gather herbs is during a sunny morning immediately after the dew dries. Avoid harvesting wet plants on damp days or in the hot sun; the plants will quickly wilt.

Walk Deliberately

You're not in a race. In fact, you're in whatever the opposite of a race is. Tread lightly. Don't walk on herbs wantonly; make your way with care so as to disturb the area as little as possible. While you're walking with a light step, keep your eyes lowered. Be aware of plants that may be hidden by other larger shrubs or covering.

At times, you'll just stop. That's right. Take a good look around, not only for the plants but to enjoy your surroundings.

Chapter 8: Preparation of the Herbs

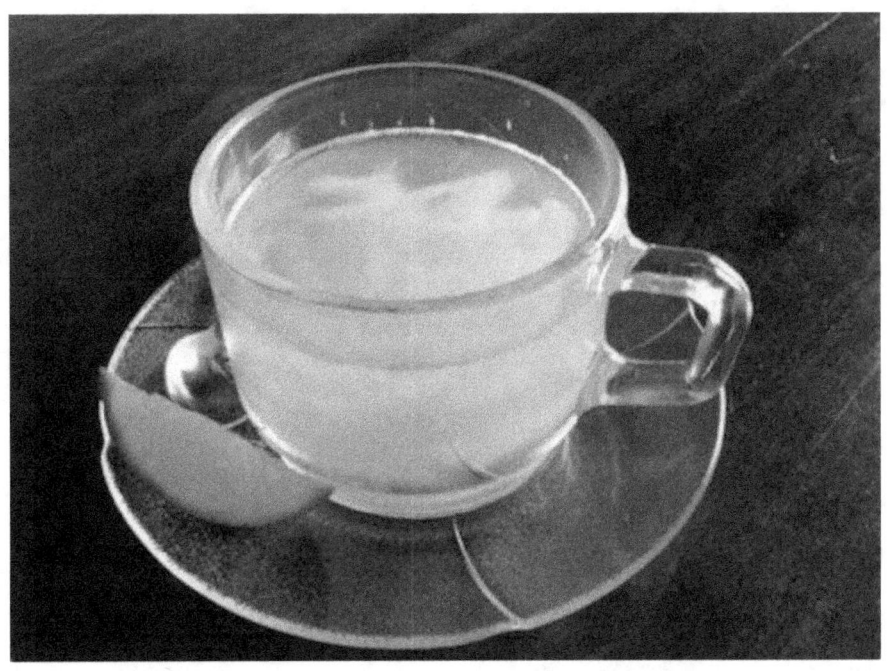

Once you have herbs home and you've prepared them, how do you use them as tools for you and your family's healing?

That's a question I'm asked frequently. If you're not already familiar with herbalists' terms, then you may naturally be confused or unsure of your next step. Many individuals' enthusiasm is dampened around this point. I don't want this to happen to you. After all, I had no idea what a poultice was when I first began, and I certainly couldn't tell you what a decoction did. It was all a mystery to me.

That's what this chapter is all about – demystifying the most common and most effective ways to use herbs, clarifying terms you may not be familiar with.

Teas

Let's start with the easiest and most familiar first. The herbal tea.

If there are no directions specific to the tea, then use a ratio of one tablespoon of dried and one teaspoon of fresh herbs for each cup of tea. The water should be freshly boiled, and there should be enough to cover all the herbs in the pot or cup. Stir the herbs to ensure they are thoroughly soaked.

Cover this during steeping. This ensures the volatile oils don't escape and you receive the tea's full medicinal strength.

Unless otherwise stated, you need to let this sit for at least 15 minutes for its full potency.

If you don't drink all the liquid, then place the remainder in a glass container (those canning jars we talked about earlier are perfect for this) and store it in the refrigerator. It will remain at its full strength for 24 hours. Any longer, the tea will not only begin to lose some of its powers, but it won't taste as good.

Not all herbs taste delicious. When that happens, you can add something to improve it. This could be honey or stevia or even freshly squeezed lemon juice.

Infusions

If you're confused about the difference between an herbal tea and an infusion, you're not alone. For the longest time, I thought they were one and the same. They both use hot water and herbs.

But there are differences, and they can be found in the number of herbs used and the steep time. An infusion uses more herbs and needs to sit for a longer time. This means that the healing potency of the infusion may be greater than that of the tea.

Most commonly, an infusion is made by the quart, as opposed to tea, which is usually brewed by the cup. You'll need about one ounce of the herb for each quart (this is where you get to use your kitchen scale). If you don't have a scale, you'll need between 4 to 12 tablespoons of herbs.

Pour hot water over this and allow it to steep overnight. If you find you need to use it sooner, allow it to sit for at least several hours. As you probably can guess, the longer it steeps, the stronger the herbal potency. To experience the drink's maximum potency, drink it within 24 hours.

To make a cold infusion, just substitute cold water. Place the mixture in the refrigerator, and be sure you allow it to steep overnight.

Decoction

If you're new to the world of herbs, you may think a decoction is merely slang for anything you mix together. But herbalism it's another form of preparing herbal remedies. It's similar to teas and infusions in that you use liquid – usually water – to extract the phytonutrients from the plant. It differs from those preparations in that a decoction is made from the plant's roots, barks, and seeds. A decoction needs to simmer longer than the other two preparations in order to ensure all the phytonutrients have been extracted.

The only thing you need to remember, that unlike teas, decoctions always use cold water initially.

Generally speaking, you'll use about one teaspoon to one tablespoon of the ground roots, barks, and seeds for each cup of cold water. Because fresh herbs contain more water than dried herbs, double the amount when you use fresh. The plant's natural moisture can dilute the strength of the decoction.

Add both the herbs and water at the same time to the pot and bring it to a gentle boil. Do not add the herbs to the boiling water. This inhibits the extraction of the phytonutrients. Then, cover the pan. Allow it to simmer for at least twenty minutes and no longer than forty. You can tell when the decoction is completed when you have about half of the liquid you started with.

Strain and transfer the liquid to individual jars, being sure to label them with identification and the date the decoction was created.

Tincture

An herbal tincture is an herb in a concentrated, liquid form. Most often, it's taken a few drops at a time, as it's placed under the tongue.

It's an effective method, but it does take preparation and resting time. Think long-term when if you're interested in healing by tincture. It will be several weeks before you can use it. But tinctures are useful, so they're worth the effort.

Tinctures are the epitome of the phrase less is more. You receive more herbal phytonutrients through several drops of tinctures than you would through a cup of tea. And you receive them faster. Your body assimilates the substance more quickly.

This method is also more convenient. If you don't have the time or patience to drink a cup of herbal tea, you can receive the same benefits from the tincture. If you are uncomfortable with placing the liquid under your tongue, you can place it in a glass of water or a cup of tea.

Yes, the tincture takes longer to prepare, but it also has an incredibly long shelf life than herbs – either fresh or dried. A tincture can last for up to five years – sometimes longer – with all of its potency preserved.

A tincture can be made from just about any part of the plant that you would use in any other form of preparation. This includes the leaves (either dried or fresh), bark, roots, and berries.

Tincture Directions:

Gather the parts of the herb you're using. Wash them and coarsely chop them. If you have a mortar and pestle, this would be the perfect time to use it. Place four ounces of the herb in a canning jar. To this, add a pint of 80 proof vodka or any other type of grain alcohol. This form of alcohol is the best extractor of the medicinal properties. If you prefer, you may use apple cider vinegar, but your tincture won't last as long.

Seal the jar and allow it to sit in a cool, dark place, and allow the magic to happen. During the first week, shake the jar daily to ensure the healing properties are evenly distributed. From the second week to the sixth, shake it about once a week.

You should allow this to sit for at least six weeks; after that, you can strain the mixture. If you have a wine press, you can use that, but it's not necessary. A cheesecloth works just fine. Just be sure you move the cloth occasionally, so you drain all the liquid.

You can also use a potato ricer to strain the tincture (I told you it would come in handy). Empty the contents of the jar into the basket of the ricer, and it does the rest. Place the resulting tincture in an airtight dark-colored glass container.

A word of advice: Don't forget to label it. Put not only what herbal tincture it is, but what parts of the plants you used and whether they were dried or fresh. Also, put the date you first made it. You may also want to label it with the proper usage.

Poultice

A poultice is a paste made of herbs bound together with water or oil that you apply topically. It's the perfect natural healing tool for external use. A poultice can be as simple as a leaf you crush by hand and place on an insect bite, and secured with a bandage.

They can be used either hot or cold. The heat increases the circulation in the affected area and draws out or removes an abscess. The cold variety is great at alleviating pain and reducing inflammation.

I'll show you two different ways of making this essential herbal healing tool. The first one is to coarsely chop the designated herbs. For this, you can use your mortar and pestle, or if you want to, you can use a food chopper or processor.

Put about two to three tablespoons of the herb (you can use more depending on the size of the area affected) in a bowl. Cover with just enough water to form a paste. I like to add a couple of tablespoons at a time until I get the right texture. The herbs should be looking like a thick paste.

Wrap this in cheesecloth or another thin cloth as a covering. You can either apply this directly to the affected area or arrange the poultice between two layers of cloth before applying it to the area. Leave it on for at least twenty minutes and up to three hours. Repeat this procedure as necessary.

Sock Poultice

If you're in need of a quick poultice, there's an easy way to apply the herb. Get a clean white cotton sock; place the chopped herbs in it and tie the top. Soak the sock in a sink or bowl of hot water. Then you're ready to apply it.

Sometimes you can put the paste directly on the wound without any cloth between the poultice and the skin. Then wrap it with anything from gauze, muslin, or even plastic wrap to keep it in place.

Dried Powders

Dried powder herbs are another method of receiving a plant's healing properties. Sometimes, a tea formula or recipe calls for it. Some individuals prefer to put powdered herbs into capsules and take them this way. Empty capsules may be bought online if you think you're interested in this.

You may also want to add herbs prepared this way to your body powder or even your toothpaste.

The one drawback to this method is that they tend to lose their potency quickly. This means you need to use them quickly and not let them sit around.

Creating powdered herbs is easy, and you've probably already guessed how to do it. Make sure the herbs are dry before putting them in a spice grinder. Grind only a small amount at a time, about one tablespoon or so. This way, you'll be sure to get everything ground small enough. Some herbalists use a mortar and pestle, but a grinder goes faster and creates a nice powdery substance.

From there, you can use them in any fashion you need them.

I've mentioned they don't keep well, but you can extend their potency by storing them in airtight containers and tucking them away in a cool place. Don't store them in direct light or in a humid location.

Infused erbal Oil

Infused oil, better known as an essential oil, is an excellent naturally topical method of easing nearly any pain you have, from sore muscles to a headache. This may be the alternative if you find pastes and poultices too messy or cumbersome. Of course, you can buy essential oils, but they're expensive, and you can never be confident of the quality of the ingredients or their strength.

It's actually quite easy to make your own infused oil and, on top of that, you have two methods from which to choose. It doesn't get much better than this.

I'll introduce you first to the no-bake method, arguably the easier of the two because the sun does all the work.

Choose a clean, glass canning jar with a lid. Then fill this with the herbs you're using. Then slowly pour the oil over the herbs. Olive and sunflower oils are the best choices. You can also use almond or grapeseed oils. The life of your herbal infusion depends on the freshness of the oil, so you'll want to use the freshest you can find.

While you're pouring, move the herbs some with a knife or fork to ensure that there are no air pockets with the oil. You'll want to cover the herbs completely, right to the brim.

Put the lid on the jar and shake it some. Place it in a cool place. It will take anywhere from three to six weeks to become totally infused. In that period, you'll need to check on it occasionally and shake it to ensure even distribution.

At the end of this period, you'll need to strain the liquid with cheesecloth into your storage containers. Squeeze the cloth to get all the liquid you can. This step can be messy, so you may want to put some paper towels down on the area or strain it on a platter.

Be sure to label the containers with the type of infusion as well as the date it was made. Generally speaking, infused herbal oils are good for up to a year if stored at room temperature. Grace always added vitamin E to her oils. It's a natural preservative and doubled the infusion's shelf-life.

If the idea of waiting a month and a half for some healing is unsettling, there's another quicker procedure that takes a day. Your crockpot. Place the herbs in your slow cooker and cover them with oil. Allow them to infuse for approximately eight hours on the low setting. Then strain into your storage bottles.

Salves and Balms

These terms are interchangeable for an herbal mixture applied topically. The herbs are combined with oils and waxes to create a pliable, soft substance. One of the interesting facts about salves and balms is they contain no water. At first glance, this may not seem to be of any importance. But, because of these, they have a long shelf life, preservative-free.

Balms and salves can be used as a topical healer for many

conditions, including sore muscles, minor cuts and scrapes, rashes, sunburn, dry, cracked skin, and even bruises.

Making these may seem intricate because it's a two-step process and requires several ingredients. But, if you have infused herbal oil on hand, you've already completed the first step. If not, follow the instructions found in that section. Then you'll continue to the next step.

If you use the ratios indicated here, you'll have about 9 ounces of herbal salve. Using a double boiler, mix 8 ounces of your choice of herbal oil with one ounce of beeswax. Heat, occasionally stirring, until the wax is melted. This is basically your balm. Dip a spoon into the mixture to ensure it's to the consistency of your liking.

You can adjust the ratios to end up with one that suits you. For a softer salve, add more oil, several drops at a time, until you find the perfect texture. For a firmer salve, add more beeswax in small chunks.

Then to be doubly sure, take a spoonful of this mixture and place it in the freezer for several minutes to get an example of what the final consistency will be. You can still make adjustments once the salve has cooled.

While the mixture is still warm, pour it into containers. These can be old jam jars or even small metal tins. Stir this with a clean fork or stick before placing the lids on the containers. Label them with the herb and date them. Once they harden, they're ready for use.

Store them in a dark, cool place. They have a shelf-life of up to a year.

Syrup

An herbal syrup is a great-tasting way to enjoy the healing benefits of not-so-great-tasting herbs. It's composed of a concentrated decoction of an herb and honey or sugar. Some people add alcohol. But the most important ingredient is the herb.

The great taste and soothing application aren't its only benefits. The honey is more than just a thickening agent; it's also a preservative. An herbal syrup has a longer shelf life than many other preparations.

Don't dismiss this method because you think it's too involved a project for you. Because it isn't. You'll find it quite a simple process. The basic instructions are simple. It's a simple 2:1 ratio: two parts herbal decoction to one part honey or sugar.

You may find some herbal authorities who prefer to use one cup herbal decoction to one cup of sugar. This extends the shelf life of the syrup, but it also increases its sweetness. If you like the sweeter taste, this is the formula you might want to use.

If you create your syrup using honey, you can expect it to have a shelf life of approximately three months. A sugar-based syrup, however, can last up to six months.

If you want to extend the life of the remedy even longer, by adding a quarter cup of alcohol for each cup of syrup.

How to Make Syrup:

Place your decoction and honey in a pan over very low heat to dissolve the honey. Be careful that the honey doesn't reach a boil. If you use sugar, you can allow this to boil gently for about 30 minutes to thicken the syrup.

Remove it from the heat. If you're adding alcohol, do so now. Pour the syrup into clean, sterile labeled bottles. Be sure not only to include the herb or herbal mixture used but the date of creation.

Store the herbal syrup in the refrigerator.

An average serving of the syrup is one-half teaspoon to one teaspoon taken one to three times daily. But of course, this also depends on the herbs you used, the person taking it, and the individual's condition and symptoms.

Chapter 9: How to Store and Dry Plants

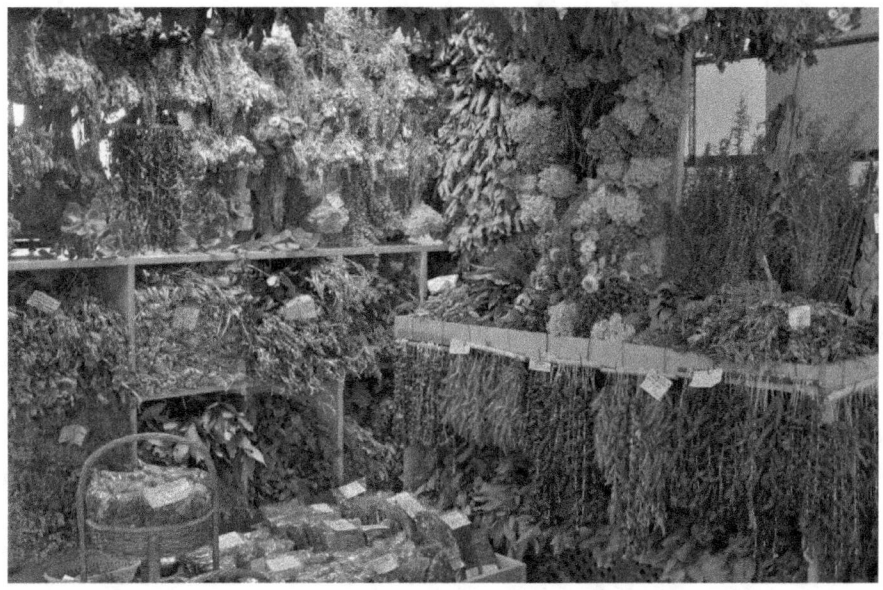

Of course, you want to enjoy the healing benefits of herbs year-round. If you're wildcrafting, this may be difficult. The next best thing is to dry the fresh herbs for the offseason.

You can even do this with the plants in your outdoor herb garden. It's the perfect way to preserve the potency of the herb, and it's easy. But the best part is that you have several methods at your fingertips.

The first and oldest method of drying fresh herbs is to tie a group of fresh plants together and hang them upside down with the leaves facing down. You should bundle between four to six stems together using either string or a rubber band. The herbs will shrink during the drying process, which means the rubber band's hold around them will loosen. As you check on your herbs during the process, be sure to look at the rubber band, as well.

Wrap them loosely in a thin paper bag of muslin in order to keep the dust off of them. The wrapping also catches the falling leaves. Don't use plastic bags because you risk the creation of mold.

Place these in a dark, cool basement for up to ten days. Check on their progress after the second week, and then weekly until they're thoroughly dried. Sometimes, it may only take seven days, depending on the size of the plants and the humidity.

When you can crush the leaves, and they sound crisp cornflakes, they're dried.

It's simple. It's quick. It's effective.

If you live in an apartment or a home with no basement, this method isn't feasible. That doesn't mean, though, you have to abandon that thought of drying fresh herbs. There are several other means to accomplish this.

Air or Rack Drying

This method involves the use of a drying rack. There racks available for purchase, especially for this purpose but, you can also make your own. Get a wooden frame and fasten muslin, cheesecloth, or netting over it. Space your herbs out on it and place them in an airy area without direct sunlight. Turn the leaves often to make sure that they're drying evenly. Within a week to ten days, your herbs should be dry.

Microwave Drying

Using a microwave can speed the process up. But you have to be careful. To do this, separate the leaves of your herbs from the stems. Wash those parts you're drying. Once the herbs have dried, place them between two paper towels and microwave them for one minute initially. Check on their progress and, if needed, continue the process for 30 seconds at a time.

It's easy to over-dry them this way. But, if you're lacking the room required for the other methods, this can work.

Drying by Dehydration

If you have a home dehydrator, this method works wonders when you need to dry herbs in bulk. Form a single layer of herbs on each of your trays, then cook them at the lowest setting for two to four hours. Be careful when you remove them; this can get tricky. You'll want to do over a clean cloth or a large bowl so you can save all the small broken herbs.

Oven Drying

If any or all of these ways sounds too complicated, then there's one other way to ensure you have a stash of dried herbs during the winter months. Look no further than your oven and a cookie sheet or baking pan. Line the pan with cheesecloth or muslin so the leaves won't stick. If you have silicone mats, that's even better. Place the heat on the lowest setting – for most ovens, this is about 170 degrees – and leave the door open a crack. Let them dry for about 30 minutes. Check on them. If the herbs aren't thoroughly, leave them in another five or ten minutes, but look in on them frequently.

While this method works, it's not the one that produces the best product. That's why I wanted until last to mention it. But, if you have no other way of drying herbs fast, then it's worth a try.

How to Store Dried Herbs

Just as you buy a glass bottle of dried herbs at the grocery, this is the best way to store home-dried herbs. You can save up old bottles or jelly jars (all cleaned well, of course) and use those, or find an airtight plastic container. The latter might not look as good, but it works just as well. When storing, decide if you want to save the whole leaf or crumble it up. For some items such as basil or mint, it's easiest to crush the leaves. The benefit of keeping the leaves whole is you get a little more fragrance when you crush them as needed.

Whole leaves also stay fresh longer. Many herbalists prefer this method, and then they grind the herbs as they need them. This is the method Grace taught me, and it's worked well.

The first rule of storage is not to allow them to sit in direct sunlight. This, of course, means your nice-looking containers aren't meant to sit on your kitchen windowsill as décor. For this reason, you may want to consider using dark-colored or tinted glass.

Your dried herbs will retain their potency longer if they are kept in a cool and dry location. You don't want these jars to sit over the stove or any place with high humidity. A root cellar is the ideal storage area, but how many of us have one? Choose the coolest room in your home or apartment, even if that means the herbs aren't in the kitchen.

Don't forget to label the containers. This may seem like obvious advice, but I've slipped several times, thinking I would remember what herb that jar held and when I dried it. More often than not, I couldn't recall. Labeling your containers is a good habit to develop.

Label the bottle with as much information as you can. In addition to the name of the herb (or herbs), list its botanical name as well. Provide the date you harvested the plant or if you don't know that the date the drying process was completed. Also, put an expiration date on it as well, so there will be no questions. This last piece of data has been very helpful to me.

Conclusion

Congratulations on your initial steps to practicing personal herbalism. I hope they won't be your last. With more than fifty herbs and more than forty ailments, this volume is a good start on your exploration of herbal healing.

The world of medicinal herbs offers you and your family a new, natural world of healing. As you progress in your journey, I hope you discover you can reduce your reliance on harsh prescription drugs. Of course, this change won't happen overnight. Nor should it. But even substituting one herb for one over-the-counter tablet is a step in the right direction.

One of the many benefits I've found that occurs when you use herbs was the increase in my general wellbeing. While my physical health improved, so did my overall happiness, my satisfaction with life, and even my relationship to a more spiritual outlook.

Regardless of the reasons you're interested in herbalism,

you'll discover an overall improvement in your life. That's one of the marvelous side-effects of holistic healing. The intent of your specific therapy with that one herb or combination of herbs may not have been to make you feel better emotionally; nonetheless, it happened.

This small volume is only a fraction of the herbal knowledge accumulated. As you progress on your journey, you'll find the information you need at just the right time. Remember, though, that if you choose this path, the travels through the herbal world is every bit important, if not more so, than the destination.

Try not to ask the question, "Am I there yet?" Rather, ask, "How much more can I learn?" Because there's also something more you can learn, whether from field guides, from veteran herbal healers, or from the plants themselves.

Grace held the traditional Native American view that all of nature is our friend. If you make friends out of the herbs you use, you'll always discover they're ready to provide you with a little bit more information.

Thank you for allowing me to share my love of herbs. My goals were simple. Not only did I want you to discover and fall in love with the healing powers of herbs. I also wanted you to fall in love with the way Grace considered them and used them. I hope I succeeded, and you're on an exciting path to wellness and holism with Native American herbs.

Appendix: Glossary

Allicin - the compound produced by chopping or crushing garlic, which provides healing benefits.

Allopathic medicine – the form of medicine in which medical health professionals treat symptoms and diseases with drugs and surgery. Sometimes called conventional medicine.

Antibiotic – any substance, natural or synthetic, that kills bacteria. Many herbs have natural antibiotic characteristics.

Antioxidant – any substance, such as vitamin C, which protects a body's cells from damage caused by unstable molecules produced during the natural metabolic process of oxidation. Free radicals are associated with the diseases and disorders associated with the aging process, including cancer and heart disease.

Antiseptic – any substance, natural or synthetic, which

prevents the spread of disease.

Antiviral agent – any substance that either destroys or suppresses the reproduction of a virus.

Ayurveda – Literally meaning "science of life" in Sanskrit, it is the traditional Hindu system of medicine, built upon the concept of holistic health.

Balm – a topical herbal application to relieve a condition. Used interchangeably with the term salve.

Beeswax – the natural substance bees secrete, which herbalists use in creating salves and balms.

Botanical – adjectival form of botany, the branch of science that studies plants.

Cardiovascular system – the body's system of blood transportation made up of the heart, arteries, capillaries, and veins.

Carrier – a substance, like an oil or beeswax, that aids in the application of an herbal remedy.

Cheesecloth – a loosely woven cotton cloth originally used to wrap cheese. Used by herbalists to strain herbs.

Dream catcher – a Native American protective talisman in the form of a framed net decorated with feathers and beads created to trap nightmares.

Drying rack – any appliance where you can lay herbs for periods of time to be air-dried undisturbed.

Expectorant – any substance, natural or synthetic, which promotes the expulsion of mucus from air passages and is used to treat coughs.

Forage- the act of searching the environment for plants to be used as food and healing herbs.

Glucose – the blood's primary sugar and the major source of the body's energy. A disruption in the control of glucose leads to a number of conditions, including diabetes.

Harvest – the process of gathering herbs for use later.

Herbalism – the study and/or practice of plants for therapeutic and medicinal purposes, usually as a form of alternative medicine.

Holistic – when referred to as an approach to medicine, the concept that treatment or therapy should take into consideration of the entire person, as opposed to simply treating the symptom.

Hypertension – high blood pressure, which exerts an excessive amount of force against the walls of your blood vessels. Hypertension increases the work your heart and blood vessels must do and may lead to the formation of plaque on the walls of the arteries and, if not treated, hardening of the arteries.

Infused oils – a carrier oil that has been permeated with either one or more herbs.

Infusion – any drink or extract prepared through the method of soaking the leaves of a plant in a liquid for healing purposes.

Metaphysical – literally meaning "beyond physics," refers many times to the spiritual realm of concepts.

Mortar and pestle – tools used by pharmacists and herbalists to grind herbs. The pestle is the heavy, blunt tool. The mortar the container in which the herbs are ground.

Muslin - a lightweight cotton cloth that is used by many herbalists used interchangeably with cheesecloth to strain herbs.

Native Americans – the indigenous peoples of what is now the continental United States, who practiced a holistic approach to all living things.

Opiate – a substance, either natural or synthetic, which dulls the senses and relieves pain. Pharmaceutical opiates are extremely strong and usually addictive.

Penicillin – an antibiotic made from the creation of certain molds. Today, the substance is created synthetically.

Phytonutrients – the natural chemicals or compounds produced by plants required by the human body for good health and the prevention of diseases.

Poultice – a mass of herbs, usually wrapped in a cloth, spread on a portion of the body for the purpose of applying moist heat as a pain-reliever or as an antiseptic.

Taproot – the largest, dominant root of a plant from which smaller roots sprout from. It is straight, thick, and tapered and always grows directly downward.

Salicin – the substance in the bark of several willows which is the precursor to salicylic acid.

Salicylic acid – an anti-inflammatory agent used in aspirin.

Salve – any ointment used to aid the healing process of the skin.

Smudge stick – a bundle of dried herbs used by the Native Americans as part of their healing ceremonies and rituals. When burnt, these herbs produce an aroma, which was said to cleanse, locations, objects, and people.

Sweat lodge – a Native American dome-shaped hut used in ritual steam baths for purification.

Synergy – the interaction of two or more substances that produces an effect greater than could have been realized by the sum of their separate actions.

Tincture – a solution of an herb or herbs in a solution of alcohol with the intent of healing.

Totem – an object normally, an animal or plant,

employed by Native Americans, which represents the powers of nature and holds spiritual significance.

Vision quest – a supernatural experience practiced by Native Americans, with the intent to interact with a guardian spirit to gain healing, advice, or protection.

Volatile oils – any oil which evaporates easily, as in essential oils.

Wildcrafting – the harvesting of herbs from their natural habitats with regard to the balance of the ecosystem. It involves the collection of only the minimal number of plants needed for one's purpose to ensure the continued growth of the plant community for the future.

www.ingramcontent.com/pod-product-compliance
Lightning Source LLC
Chambersburg PA
CBHW070325220526
45467CB00001B/40